T0188607

Digital Health Promotion

Digital Health Promotion
A Critical Introduction

Ivy O'Neil

polity

First published in 2019 by Polity Press

Polity Press
65 Bridge Street
Cambridge CB2 1UR, UK

Polity Press
101 Station Landing
Suite 300
Medford, MA 02155, USA

ISBN-13: 978-1-5095-3330-5
ISBN-13: 978-1-5095-3331-2 (pb)

A catalogue record for this book is available from the British Library.

Library of Congress Cataloging-in-Publication Data

Names: O'Neil, Ivy, author.
Title: Digital health promotion : a critical introduction / Ivy O'Neil.
Description: Cambridge, UK ; Medford, MA : Polity Press, 2019. | Includes
   bibliographical references and index.
Identifiers: LCCN 2019007298 (print) | LCCN 2019007857 (ebook) | ISBN
   9781509533336 (Epub) | ISBN 9781509533305 (hardback) | ISBN 9781509533312
   (pbk.)
Subjects: | MESH: Health Promotion | Health Information Management | Medical
   Informatics | Public Health
Classification: LCC R858 (ebook) | LCC R858 (print) | NLM WA 590 | DDC
   362.10285--dc23
LC record available at https://lccn.loc.gov/2019007298

Typeset in 11 on 13 pt Sabon by
Servis Filmsetting Ltd, Stockport, Cheshire
Printed and bound in Great Britain by CPI Group (UK) Ltd, Croydon

For further information on Polity, visit our website: politybooks.com

Contents

Detailed Contents

Acknowledgements

I would like to thank Polity's editorial and production team, Jonathan Skerrett and Karina Jákupsdóttir, for their help throughout the production of this book. Also thanks to the reviewers who reviewed the book proposal and the final draft. Their comments and suggestions have been valuable.

I would also like to thank Leeds Beckett University for the use of library resources and for my experience and friendship gained throughout my career as Principal Lecturer in the Health Promotion team.

Thanks to my previous students Vitalis Mwinyuri and Mzwandile Mpongwana for providing me with practice examples of using digital technology in the health promotion field in their country.

To my friends and family, particularly to Alex, Alasdair and Cat, a very special thanks for their tolerance, support and encouragement throughout the course of writing this book. Finally, a special thanks to Cat who illustrated the book cover. Thank you.

Acknowledgements

1

Introduction

This chapter provides an introduction to the topic area, the rationale for the book and an outline of the areas to be covered in relation to the development and the practical uses of digital technologies in promoting health; the underpinning health promotion theories; the Big Data phenomenon; tackling and managing public health issues and improving health outcomes. The chapter will introduce the reader to digital technology within a behaviour approach to health promotion and its potential effects on health inequalities. An explanation will be given regarding the organization of the book. A chapter-by-chapter introduction of its content will also be given to point readers to specific chapters. The book focuses specifically on public health and health promotion and will not cover technological developments in acute secondary healthcare.

This book is primarily for postgraduate-level students studying public health and health promotion, and final-year students at undergraduate level in all health-related courses. It is also useful for students on a professional course such as medicine, nurses, public health practitioners, professions allied to health and environmental health, primary care, practitioners in a wide range of health and social care environments who are interested in health promotion, as well as anyone with a role in health improvements. Because of the connectivity of digital technologies, the sharing of the complex web of information and the Big Data phenomenon, the impacts of eHealth development spread out broadly and globally. Therefore, this book would be useful for students and practitioners both in the UK and internationally. The implications of neoliberalism are particularly relevant for a 'westernized / Global North' policy context, such as in the USA, Canada, European countries or Australia. Many of the examples are from the Global South (particularly Africa) and the underlying health promotion principles are, and should be, global.

It is inevitable that technology will develop beyond the publication of this text. This book is not primarily intended as a 'best apps' or 'how to' manual, guiding readers in using current digital applications. It is about becoming Health Promotion literate regarding digital technologies. The crucial element is about teasing out the health promotion principles and underpinning theories to be applied to digital health technology as it develops. The intention is to be able to assess *future* as well as *current* developments in a way that gives us confidence to critique and become better informed in the use of new technologies as they emerge.

Digital technology – an unprecedented series of developments

The realities of digital technological change are a part of everyday life, both in technological advancement and in societal behaviours. In 1994, the internet in the UK was only used by 0.5% of the population. By 2014, 84% had internet access, and 76% accessed the internet every day (Office for National Statistics 2014). People over 65 increasingly use the internet, rising from 9% in 2006 to 42% in 2014 (Ofcom 2014). Approximately four in five UK households have fixed broadband, and three in five adults access the internet through their mobile phone. In 2015, 68% of adults aged 75+ would miss having a TV set in their home as compared to 17% of 16- to 24-year-olds. However, 59% of those aged 16–24 are more likely to miss their mobile phone, as compared with just 2% of those aged 75+ (Ofcom 2015). The use of tablets and smartphones continues to increase. However, there are still 12% of people unable to use the internet and some with no plans for future use (Coulter and Mearns 2016).

In the USA, 79% of online adults use the internet, and half of older adults have home broadband and 42% reportedly own a smartphone (PEW 2016). According to Burke-Garcia and Scally (2014), internet use is fairly broadly distributed across race, gender, income and education. However, a study by Duggan and Brenner in the USA in 2012 shows that women, people from urban settings and people under 50 are more likely to use social networking sites, particularly those aged 18–29 (83%, as against 32% of the 65+). Similarly, there are more young people and people in urban areas who use Twitter. Young people and women, as well as African Americans and Hispanics, are also more likely to use Instagram. Facebook, however, remains the most popular social networking site for younger people aged 18–29 (86%, as against 35% of the 65+), and for women more than men (72%, against 62%) (Duggan and Brenner 2013). According to Mark Zuckerberg, founder and CEO at Facebook, as from June 2017, there are officially 2 billion people on Facebook, the biggest online social networking site globally (PEW 2016), and 1.5 billion users on YouTube, the second-most-used search engine in the world (Techcrunch 2017). This sets a context for the potential importance of digital technologies in health. Chapter 2 will provide a critical review of the current usage of digital technology in the public health arena.

Communicating health

With the rapid pace of development, digital technologies offer a wide range of potential influences on health and health behaviours. Increased usages of social media (for example, among young people and ethnic minority groups) make such sites a potentially good channel for health communication. It is also useful for sharing health messages among friends and families in social groups in a speedy manner. Web 2.0 technology with its specific interactive functionality offers new dimensions for health communications such as interpersonal communication, narrowcasting and tailored messaging (Atkin and Rice 2013). Views and information can be shared in blogs, podcasts, via Twitter, interactive video, Instagram, WhatsApp and many social networking sites such as Facebook; narrowcasting via audience segmentation can be used in social marketing strategies via media campaigns; tailored messages can be sent to target audiences via text messaging; data can also be tracked and used for large-scale research (Ofcom 2015). Interpersonal communication can be improved via online mentors and email. Health messages can be put on online banners (Atkin and Rice 2013). New technology to improve efficiency of service provision is being seen as a solution in the age of austerity when funding is limited. However, many people who lack access to the internet or the required skills may not be able to benefit from the advance of technology.

For example, in the UK, efforts to digitize the healthcare system have been ongoing and can be dated back to the 1960s, with the first national information technology (IT) strategy for the NHS in 1992 (NHS Management Executive 1992). Connecting for Health was a strategy aimed at creating a single electronic health record for patients, connecting primary and secondary care IT systems, providing a single platform for health professionals. Almost all general practices in England were using electronic health records by mid-2000 (Wachter 2016). Progress was made in the 2000s particularly in primary care, whereas secondary care lagged behind significantly (National Audit Office 2013). In England in 2013, the Secretary of State for Health challenged the NHS to 'go paperless' by 2018, with the publication of the *NHS Five Year Forward View* in 2014 (subsequently extended to 2020). The National Information Board (2014) set out to enable people to make the right health and care choices through full access to their care records, access to the use of health and care apps and digital information services. Care professionals and carers should also have access to all the data, information and knowledge they need by 2020 for quality care provision, supporting research and ensuring cost-effectiveness through the use of technology. Its report *Personalised Health and Care: A Framework for Action 2020* (National Information Board 2014) set out the implementation plan aimed at improving 'digital maturity'. Funding was set aside to meet this challenge. Recommendations were also made by the Wachter review (2016) to digitize secondary care. It was proposed all Health Trusts should achieve 'digital maturity' by 2023.

The development of modern health technology is swift. Clearly, there are potential benefits in the use of technology to improve healthcare. Care services can be better planned and co-ordinated. More effective and efficient services can be provided by healthcare professionals. People can take a more active role in and control of their own health and care (Klasnja and Pratt 2012). Cyberspace can be an effective platform for health promotion. However, as we will discuss in the coming chapters, there is still a lack of research on the use of social media in the public health field (Burke-Garcia and Scally 2014). The quality and accuracy of internet information, as well as data security, are of concern (Ahmad et al. 2006; Hou and Shim 2010; Ratzan 2011). The NHS-HE Forum Connectivity Best Practice Working Group identified risks in the use of social media, including confidentiality, ownership issues and cyberbullying (Lafferty 2013).

Drawing information together, Gretton and Honeyman (2016) from The King's Fund looked at new developing technologies, identifying eight technologies, with examples from both the UK and the USA, that will change health and care, making it more effective, efficient and sophisticated in modern-day healthcare provision:

1 **The smartphone** – a mobile device with internet connectivity and computing ability, sensors for tracking health data and many downloadable health apps. It can serve as the hub for diagnostic and health management technology, e.g. management of type 1 diabetes.
2 **At-home or portable diagnostics** – devices and apps such as portable X-ray machines, blood-testing kits, the AliveCor Heart monitor and Alive ECG app. Smart assistive technology can be accessed and used at home to assess and monitor patients' progress, e.g. in Parkinson's disease or asthma.
3 **Smart or implantable drug delivery mechanisms** – implanted drug delivery devices can be used to deliver medications, monitor drug compliance – e.g., via smart pills – and help people with long-term conditions such as dementia or Parkinson's disease.
4 **Digital therapeutics** – digital therapy platforms that can connect people with their peers and health professionals in the management of long-term conditions, e.g. computerized cognitive behavioural therapy. Preventative interventions such as lifestyle coaching and group therapy can be used in the prevention of chronic conditions, e.g. diabetes.

5 **Genome sequencing** – a new technology such as nanopore technology can help to improve understanding of the development of illness and its treatment in an individual. Population-level genome data can also be collected to understand population health.

6 **Machine learning** – a type of artificial intelligence that enables a computer to learn and make sense of large amounts of unstructured data for health service provision.

7 **Blockchain technology** – a decentralized database can be used (for example) in improving existing electronic health records. One of the most well-known applications in this area is the digital currency Bitcoin.

8 **The connected community** – internet space has become a venue for people from across the world to meet, support and share information with each other.

However, all the above are still overly focused on service-centred usages and, as this book will discuss, the concept of health and health improvement is much broader. In this book, we will explore in more depth the meaning of health and healthcare in the context of public health, look more fundamentally at health and digital developments, and discuss the nature and wider impacts of digital technologies on health.

Overview and rationale of the book

In the short space of a decade, the development of digital technology has radically and unimaginably reshaped our world, and continues to impact on our lives. We have become technologically dependent on the use of interactive technologies in modern living (Gold et al. 2012; Atkin and Rice 2013; Capurro et al. 2014; Lupton 2015c), and particularly so for young people (Centre for Health Promotion, Women's and Children's Health Network 2012; Loss et al. 2014). Within health fields, modern technologies can potentially enhance health services provision, increasing accessibility, effectiveness and efficiency, both on healthcare provision and in the management of healthcare services. We have seen examples of this in terms of organizations such as the English NHS going paperless (Department of Health 2013b), and the Scottish

Government committing to a world-class digital service (Scottish Government 2013). The transformation of health and social care is about empowering everyone to live longer and healthier. Health-promoting services need interconnectedness for efficient and effective service provision.

The use of social media and electronic communication technologies in tackling public health issues is increasingly common. Internet searching for health information and the use of health apps on mobile devices can be seen as a daily activity for many. Initiatives on eHealth and mHealth, such as electronic health records, mobile telemedicine, health call centres, telephone helplines, as well as text messaging, blogs, Twitter, Facebook and telecommunication, are being used for information provision, communication and for providing support in cyberspace (Gold et al. 2012; Atkin and Rice 2013; Capurro et al. 2014). Gamification, surveillance and monitoring are widely explored for managing chronic conditions such as diabetes, and health-promoting activities, benefiting patients and professionals (Javitt 2014; Boulos et al. 2015). European countries are very active in developing mHealth (WHO 2011a). The World Health Organization (WHO) (2011a) supports the development of mobile apps (mHealth), developing databases, evaluation frameworks, and providing information on public health best practice.

With the effects of globalization and the Big Data phenomenon in an increasingly digitally 'connected' world where health information is at our fingertips, healthcare decisions are made on complex connections of information. As individuals, most of us have instant access to health information anytime anywhere, enabling us to manage and make informed choices about our health. As professionals, we make research- and evidence-based healthcare decisions and provide healthcare services based on copious amounts of information about the populations we serve. However, the improved accessibility of health information and the surveillance ability of digital technology also lead to concerns about privacy and data security issues (WHO 2011a; Lupton 2015c).

It is important to be alert to the strengths and opportunities of digital technology developments. It is also important to recognize the weaknesses and threats. Technology can be both empowering and disempowering if not used appropriately. We need to have a better understanding of the underpinning theories and be critical about how they can be used effectively. Digitized activities in tackling public health issues currently have an underlying assumption that the individual is responsible for their own health; motivation and engagement are tacitly assumed to obviously be in place for behaviour change (Lupton 2015c). All too often, the individual is assumed to be readily empowered. If health apps are available to all, it is assumed everyone will be equally likely to use them or can be encouraged to use them; if they are used, it is assumed the benefit will follow for everyone equally. Such assumptions were long ago seen as inadequate in mainstream health as this ignores the structural barriers and social determinants of health, such as education, transport, employment opportunities ... (Dixey 2013; Lupton 2013a; Baum and Fisher 2014; Cross et al. 2017). Studies on poverty already show that not everyone is readily empowered for even the most accessible approaches. We need to move beyond individualist neoliberal models in health service provision to address the structural barriers to health improvement (Cross et al. 2017). This will be explored in depth in the coming chapters.

Health promotion is about social justice, equity of health and reducing health inequalities. This is a critical and analytical text that encourages students and practitioners to understand how the underpinning theoretical and ideological perspectives of health promotion relate to digital health. It encourages students to consider the recent rapid development of digital technology; to reflect on their practice as public health practitioners and, at the management level, as public health managers and leaders; and to think informatively, critically and analytically about the applications and implications of the use of these digital technologies, and their effects on health outcomes and health inequalities, as well as health inequities. There is also a need for resources to support the use of these technologies. Not everyone has a smartphone or computer, or is proficient in using them. We already know that not everyone is equally well resourced, motivated and empowered to seek out and select healthy choices, be that online or in the real world. There is no doubt digital technology offers many opportunities for public health practice. However, there are many social, economic, political and ethical implications (Lupton 2015c). There may also be a risk of contributing to an ever-widening health inequalities gap, both within and between countries, as discussed by Marmot (Marmot 2010), and to a failure to address health promotion principles and values.

Organization of the book

This book will critique current developments of digital technologies in public health and health promotion in tackling public health issues through a Social Model perspective. It will look at the underpinning theoretical perspectives of health communication and human behaviour; the important issues of power and empowerment, as well as the need for collaboration and participation in health matters. The implications of Big Data and public health management, and the applications and usefulness of modern technology in promoting health and reducing health inequalities will be critically discussed. The book will also seek to stimulate those in health promotion activities to be critical of how present and future developments are consistent (or in conflict) with underlying health promotion principles.

The book is divided into seven chapters.

- **Chapter 1** is this introductory chapter.
- **Chapter 2** is an overview of recent developments and uses of electronic and digital technologies to promote health in practice. It will discuss some familiar technologies, such as smartphones and health apps, wearables, social media, social networking sites; and the use of digital technology in some areas of healthcare, e.g. telehealth and telecare. It will explore the concept of gamification and consider applications such as active video games and serious games. It will also discuss the use of digital technology among different population groups and in different areas of health promotion – such as among young people, in mental health, sexual health.
- **Chapter 3** will explore the concept of health and how health can be promoted, relating the principles, values and practice of health promotion to the use of digital technology. It will consider determinants of health, power, choice and control, and principles of empowerment and participation in digital health. It will also look at the use of digital platforms as a virtual setting

for health promotion, and health promotion ethics in digital health interventions.

- **Chapter 4** will discuss the emphasis of digital health in a neo-liberal environment on behavioural and lifestyle approaches to health promotion and their effectiveness, relating to underpinning behaviour theories; health practice versus health behaviour; and the continued neglect of social, economic and cultural determinants of health. It will also explore social marketing and behaviour change relating to digital health.
- **Chapter 5** will set out current issues in public health and public health management. It will explore the Big Data phenomenon; public health research and surveillance in the Big Data environment; as well as issues such as data security, privacy, confidentiality and cyberbullying.
- **Chapter 6** will discuss the importance of health policies in health promotion and in digital health, and the concepts of nudge and choice architecture. It will discuss the potential risk of digital health in the widening of health inequality and health inequity gaps. It will also look at health literacy and the digital divide as well as eHealth literacy, and the impact of digital technology among different groups of internet users.
- **Chapter 7** draws together the discussions in previous chapters, looking forward to the future use of digital technology, in research and development, as we enter into the era of Web 3.0 and the Internet of Things. The book will end with a list of recommendations on the use of digital technology.

Useful reading

The following three books are essential texts for students undertaking an M.Sc. Public Health – Health Promotion course. They are very useful to read in conjunction with this book. This will provide you with an in-depth understanding of health promotion.

Cross, R., Davis, S. and O'Neil, I. (2017) *Health Communication: Theoretical and Critical Perspectives*. Cambridge: Polity.

Dixey, R. (ed.) (2013) *Health Promotion: Global Principles and Practice*. CABI.

Green, J., Tones, K., Cross, R. and Woodall, J. (2015) *Health Promotion: Planning and Strategies*. 3rd edition. London: Sage.

2

Recent Development in Digital Technology Relating to Public Health

Key points

- To consider the conceptual landscape of digital technology in public health.
- To discuss recent developments of some familiar technologies used in health arenas, e.g. smartphones and health apps, wearables, social media, social networking sites.
- To discuss the use of digital technology in some areas of healthcare, e.g. telehealth and telecare.
- To explore the concept of gamification and consider active video games and serious games.
- To discuss the use of digital technology among different population groups and different areas of health promotion, such as young people, mental health, sexual health.

Introduction

The development of information communication technology (ICT) has grown exponentially in the past decade, in parallel with technology-based healthcare interventions, impacting on the way we communicate health messages and tackle public health issues. These include mobile phones as communication devices for text messaging (Hazelwood 2008; Head et al. 2013), for information-giving, confirming appointments, providing test results. Interactive Web 2.0 technologies, such as social media platforms, health apps and tracking technologies, can be downloaded onto smartphones for information provision, health monitoring and tracking purposes (WHO 2011a; Gold et al. 2012; Lewis et al. 2012; Piette et al. 2012; Centre for Health Promotion, Women's and Children's Health Network 2012; Atkin and Rice, 2013; Capurro et al. 2014; Loss et al. 2014; Lupton 2015c). Wearable devices such as Fitbits have become common Christmas or birthday presents for friends and relatives. Anonymity in web information helps with sensitive topics such as sexual health and mental health. The idea of game-playing (gamification) can also help to engage people in health promotion activities. Social networking sites can be used to provide social support to the public, increasing quality of life and self-efficacy (Atkin and Salmon 2010; Atkin and Rice 2013), and to help young people with mental health conditions, as well as improving relationships between patients and healthcare professionals (Martin et al. 2011).

This chapter will provide a review of the literature on the use of digital technology in recent years in different areas of public health practice. It is not a review of the current best digital health applications, nor is it a manual – not a 'how to' guide. It is intended, rather, to give a more conceptual framework on the development of digital technology and its implications, and the potential and challenges for health and healthcare.

Digital technology and health – a changing landscape

This chapter takes a timeline approach, looking at digital health from the Web 1.0 period when technology is about database information-gathering and information-provision and the computer is just a digital library, a one-way communication device, progressing to today's Web 2.0 period, where technology is about interactiveness and connectedness. Today's technology is about both the smart hardware – such as smartphones, tablets, mobile devices – and smart software, such as the sophisticated health apps, and social media, which allow feedback, providing interactive two-way communication for the users. The continuing

Box 2.1 Digital technology and health communication

		Forms of communication	Examples
Web 1.0	Direct one-way communication	Mass communication	Information provision
Web 2.0	Interactive two-way communication	Interpersonal communication	Text messaging
		Mass communication	Twitter, blogs
Web 3.0	Interactive two-way communication	Communicate between people and between machines. Has the ability to interpret, organize data into meaningful information and perform tasks.	Artificial intelligence Tracking daily activities and suggesting health promotion actions.

present timeline of Web 3.0 – such as the Internet of Things, and Artificial Intelligence (AI) technology – will be considered in the last chapter, looking forwards to the future.

Twenty years ago, new technology's place was within IT departments developing management information systems and relational databases, helping organizations to be smart, joined-up and paperless. It was about enhancing the conventional usages of media – newsprint, television, radio, cinema ... New technology was mainly for communication, information provision, record keeping ... The mobile phone was just 'a phone'; 'innovation' was about being able to individualize your phone with a different-coloured clip-on fascia. Usage started to broaden, from the everyday uses of new technology making daily life easier to the remote-controlled assistance of smart technologies in care settings.

In health terms, 20–30 years ago, digital technology was about the increase of capacity, evident in Moore's Law (1965) about the number of transistors in an integrated circuit doubling every two years. By the 1980s, these developments had reached into commercial, public-service and educational organizations – it was about enhancing and developing administrative capacities. IT was a large-scale, 'top down' investment. IT strategies were about existing processes done more cost-effectively and efficiently – payroll, information storage and retrieval. Technology began to migrate from corporate mainframe to mini- and microcomputers. The need was to manage the complexity of data within organizations – Big Data did not exist. The mobile phone was a tool provided by and for the workplace. The improvement of technology began to widen to the delivery of services in the last ten years. Mobile phones were used for service provision such as text messaging. Care was about developing smart homes and smart technology for older and disabled people.

The landscape of today's digital technology is more complex:

- Corporations and public services still invest in major new digital technology. But the corporate interest has expanded beyond the 'internal' organizational capability to the much more societal and commercial 'Big Data' reality.
- Technology has become much more affordable and consumers have rapidly become key players through their purchasing power.
- The technology itself has become much more sophisticated and powerful with comprehensive health applications.
- There is an interplay between individualism, consumerism, globalization and neoliberalism. Consumers are citizens and all citizens are co-equal consumers. The question becomes who is entitled and who is excluded?
- There are major questions about what actually has an impact. Does the 'digital technology' produce a sustained change in behaviour leading to an equally sustained improvement in health?
- Digital developments are also about the harm they may cause in areas such as data security, privacy and confidentiality and cyberbullying.

New digital technologies are increasingly common in high-income, post-industrial countries in Europe, the USA and beyond. For example, in the USA, DeMartini et al. (2013) found a significant increase in digital access and usage in recent years among families in urban areas: 80% of the study families had internet access and 78% reported using Facebook, with more than 70% of the study families owning a smartphone. Their study demonstrated a great potential for the use of digital technologies in health communication. But it's also important to note that technologies are not simply relevant for the technologically rich Global North. In lower-income Global South countries, such as those in Africa, mobile phone coverage is above 79%. It was estimated that 85%

of the world's population had access to commercial wireless signals in 2010 (WHO 2011a). The author has been a visiting lecturer teaching health promotion in some African countries for a number of years; the increased use of mobile phones among her students was very evident over these years. The use of iPads and dongles for internet access was also increasingly a familiar sight in her African classrooms. Although internet access tends to be better in cities and in more affluent communities, the progressive use of technologies universally – for example, smartphones – is becoming commonplace.

Mobile technologies used in healthcare, including health promotion, have become a 'new field of eHealth' (WHO 2011a). While there has been a lack of evaluation of eHealth programmes at this earlier stage of eHealth development (WHO 2011a; Gold et al. 2012), there is general agreement that digital technological development has great potential for healthcare and health promotion. It may also help access populations seen as hard-to-reach. However, increased internet dependence also poses challenges, particularly in providing services for socially, economically and digitally disadvantaged groups – e.g. low-income families, disabled people, rural communities – which will be discussed in more depth in chapter 6. As discussed by many authors, disparities remain (Chou et al. 2013; Lupton 2015c; Marschang 2014; Cross et al. 2017; Ren et al. 2017). Online health information can be a useful source (Stevenson et al. 2007; Fox and Jones 2009). Hou and Shim (2010) found a high level of trust in internet health information. As digital technologies progress, Web 2.0 interactive technologies offer great potential, with the ability for two-way information exchanges – an 'indispensable communication tool' (Bennet and Glasgow 2009: 274), and a new 'setting' for health promotion (Loss et al. 2014). However, there are also barriers: inaccurate and misleading information, lack of investment, privacy and safety issues (Ren et al. 2017), which will be discussed further in chapter 5.

From Web 1.0 to Web 2.0 era – some older technologies still dominate

When we think about the use of digital technology, we tend to think of the internet, social media, smartphones ... But

lower-tech digital technologies such as television and radio transmission, important for health communication twenty years ago,
are still important for some today. These commonplace electronic
low-tech media for mass communication are particularly accessible for people with low reading skills. Television (terrestrial,
satellite and increasingly online) reaches a large audience. Radio
transmission is very important for those on the move, such as
professional drivers, outdoor workers, car travellers or populations in rural areas with poor television signals (Cross et al.
2017). Other than formal advertisements on television or radio
from health services – e.g. Drink and Drive campaigns – or
documentaries, news items, current affairs or programmes debat-
ing current issues are also important for health communication.
There are also programmes such as soap operas on television and
radio, which can be very influential. They mirror an audience's
construction of reality and focus on common concerns (Green et
al. 2015; Cross et al. 2017). Activities labelled as enter-educate,
edutainment, entertainment-education, infotainment, can also be
useful in sensitive areas such as sexual health. Audiences can be
receptive both emotionally and intellectually to these programmes
(Cross et al. 2017).

   Radio was second only to face-to-face interactions in both
urban and rural areas in many low- and middle-income countries.
Radio had widespread and low-cost advantages. One example
of the use of radio as a health communication channel comes
from one of the author's students in relation to malaria-control
campaigns for indoor residual spraying and insecticide-treated
bed nets in Ghana. An evaluation from 2012 to 2014 highlighted
radio's importance in health promotion across all eight districts
in the upper west Ghana region (Mwinyuri 2014, unpublished).
However, for an intervention that requires wide participation
from the community, one communication tool may not adequately
reach specific segments of society. A multi-pronged strategy is
more effective in mass communication (Wakefield et al. 2010).
Timing of transmission is also important to ensure delivery of
messages to everyone using mass communication media. It was
found that evening broadcasts between 6.30 p.m. and 8.30 p.m.
are most effective in reaching a wide audience. Digital technology
can reduce the cost of health promotion interventions. However,
one must be careful regarding the ethical concerns around the use

of modern technologies (Mwinyuri 2014, unpublished). This will be discussed in the next chapter.

The telephone (mobile or landline) is an important and under-used technology for healthcare delivery and for support (Coulter and Mearns 2016). In fact, telephone helplines are successful health communication channels (e.g. child abuse helplines, the Samaritans, etc.). The telephone as a basic technology has been used for providing advice and support for many years – e.g., phone advice from doctors and nurses in health services. But it has limitations. The national GP patient survey on telephone consultation suggested that preference for this type of consultation is low. Only 6 per cent of respondents said they prefer to speak to their GP on the phone, although this could be due to the lack of awareness of telephone consultation availability. Despite this, 12 per cent of consultations are actually carried out by phone and many GP practices continue to encourage telephone consultation, e.g. for patients' convenience (Coulter and Mearns 2016). A study by Campbell et al. (2014) on patients requesting same-day primary care appointments also suggested that the introduction of GP triage or nurse triage reduced face-to-face GP consultations. However, it increased the number of primary care contacts and overall workload in the 28 days after the requested appointment, e.g. from face-to-face to telephone contact, and shifting GP workload to nurses. The study showed that there was no difference in the average costs of healthcare or health outcomes associated with either form of triage, but there was an effect on patients' experience of care, e.g. reduction in patient satisfaction.

Telephone coaching can be another method for effective self-management support. Although costly, it can motivate people to adopt healthy behaviour and boost confidence (The Evidence Centre 2014). Health coaching was widespread in the USA, and is now used in the UK. Birmingham OwnHealth was an earlier example in the UK, aiming to improve self-care and reduce health service use. However, this was decommissioned following an assessment by Steventon et al. (2013) showing disappointing results. According to Coulter and Mearns (2016), the success of telephone coaching is mixed, and the reason for this was unclear. So, conventional low-tech solutions are still being used, are being developed for health improvement strategy, and they need to be evaluated comprehensively for future learning and evidence-based practice.

Some older but evolving technologies

As the use of mobile phones increases, simple text messaging using these devices has become a very common form of social communication and a cost-effective intervention. In 2011, 75 per cent of cell phone owners reported regularly sending and receiving text messages (Kohut et al. 2011). Hazelwood (2008) used a mobile phone text messaging service for her clients with eating disorders, with positive results. Health professionals could construct a careful tailored message and their clients could revisit their advice repeatedly. A meta-analysis by Head et al. (2013) found that text messaging is particularly effective when messages are tailored and personalized. Health communication using technology has become interpersonal, two-way and interactive. The investment in digital health has moved to personal use and individual focus, rather than corporate, as compared to twenty years ago. Digital development is becoming bottom-up, not top-down.

This is also true in many low-resource countries. The use of mobile phone technology and phone network coverage are expanding. For example, across Sub-Saharan Africa, the mobile phone is a valuable tool in public health. In 2010, mobile phone ownership was already at 73 per cent in a survey in South India; 66 per cent used phones to contact their health provider; weekly phone reminders also helped to facilitate medication adherence (Shet et al. 2010). In Zambia, mHealth technology can offer reliable and sustainable solutions to the slow reporting of infant HIV test results to health facilities and quicken the delivery of test results to caregivers by using text messaging. It can also help to improve antiretroviral (ART) treatment adherence through reminder calls and/or SMS messages (Shet et al. 2010; Seidenberg et al. 2012; Free et al. 2013). Free et al.'s (2013) systematic review suggested text messaging increased adherence to ART treatment in low-income countries, and smoking cessation in high-income countries. However, their findings provided mixed evidence for the effectiveness of healthcare intervention delivery. The authors also highlighted the need for high-quality controlled trials in the use of mHealth applications. Limitations in healthcare infrastructure, laboratory diagnostic capacity and healthcare staff in low-income countries are significant when good surveillance is important (for example, in the management of influenza pandemics and control of other disease outbreaks, such as malaria and diarrhoeal illness). In Madagascar, the sentinel surveillance network allows fast transmission of encrypted short messages via mobile phone, enabling daily analysis and data monitoring, facilitating fast responses for infectious disease control. Mobile phone technology is a cheap and readily available tool in healthcare; however, the costs of system maintenance, such as resources for staffing, can be high (Rajatonirina et al., 2012).

Digital and telephone advice services have also developed over the past twenty years. In the UK, for example, through the NHS Choices website or the NHS 111 telephone advice, services such as booking appointments, searching for health information, checking quality of services, and downloading self-care apps are available (Coulter and Mearns 2016). This can help people take more control of their health and care, interacting with care professionals more effectively. However, many GPs complained this increased workloads, with patients re-directed to them via internet services (Coulter and Mearns 2016). Many people look for information about diseases and symptoms on the internet (National Health Service (NHS) Choices 2015). However, considering people over 65 need health advice most, only 21 per cent of them used it for health information, and much fewer used it for any wider purpose. They didn't seem to use telephones for advice either. Coulter and Mearns (2016) suggested the reasons were lack of computer skills, lack of smartphone ownership, lack of trust in the information, and a general preference for face-to-face contacts.

Sometimes, habitual dependence on these more familiar, older technologies can hold back development of more up-to-date possibilities. Online usage for health services still lags behind commercial or other public-sector internet usages. Most GP practices still use telephone for appointment bookings (Ipsos MORI 2015). In May 2015, 97% of GPs in England offered online services such as appointment booking, prescription requests, and accessing health record summaries, compared with 32% in April 2014 (Ipsos MORI 2015). However, only 10% of patients had ordered prescriptions online, 6% had booked appointments online, and only 0.5% had accessed their online medical record. According to Coulter and Mearns (2016), availability and/or the awareness of these online services is low. Further research is needed to find reasons for low usage and ways of promoting digital services if their use is to be successful.

Reflection 2.1

Think of your own experience of the use of digital technology in health promotion, either that you have encountered as a member of the public or in your own practice? How do you think digital health interventions can enhance health promotion? And what would be the challenges?

Technological development – smartphone and health apps

Smartphones allow health-related apps to be downloaded; text, photos and videos can be sent; internet searching of health information can be used for health communication purposes. The interactivity of these technologies can offer support anytime, anywhere. Mobile phone use has become user-driven and user-determined. Health apps can help people make informed choices on their healthcare needs. They can empower people to take charge of their own health. There are around 165,000 health-related apps available via Apple's iOS and Google's Android (IMS Health 2015), with Europe and North America as the biggest markets (Deloitte 2015). The technology can be specific in its usage, with low-cost development and low-cost access. Apps for monitoring exercise, diet and weight are most popular (Fox and Duggan 2012). Bert et al. (2014) found mHealth apps increasingly used for setting up nutritional goals – e.g., by counting calories or food diaries – and physical-activity and lifestyle modification tips. Alghamdi et al. (2015) examined the opportunities and challenges of using mHealth apps in developing countries, finding that the majority of mHealth apps are used for smoking cessation, weight loss and chronic disease management.

The English NHS health apps library set up in 2013 curated the best-quality health apps. However, data security was poor (Huckvale et al. 2015). The health apps library was withdrawn in 2015 with a new apps library and health apps-appraising model, the new NHS Apps Library, beta-launched in April 2017 with apps in different areas – such as myCOPD, breast cancer, Talking

Point for dementia, Brush DJ for dental health, mumoActive for Type 1 diabetes, GDm-Health for pregnant women, Evergreen Life for personal health records – and many others downloadable through the website. There is also Mobile Health space for health apps developers developing digital products. Public feedback can help apps developers meet quality standards of safety and effectiveness (NHS 2017).

Using the data from the Health Information National Trend Survey in an American study on the use of mHealth apps among US adults, Bhuyan et al. (2016) found that people who had mHealth apps tended to be younger, married, have a higher education level and a higher annual household income, live in urban areas, have health insurance coverage, be more confident in looking after their own health, and have fewer comorbidities. They reported that these findings are reflected in the wider literature. Among their sample of adults who had smartphones or tablets, 36% had mHealth apps on their device; of these, 60% reported usefulness in achieving health behaviour goals, and 35% for medical care decision making. Krebs and Duncan (2015) also found that 52.8% of their study participants reported that they used health apps for tracking physical activity, 47.6% tracking what they eat and 46.8% tracked weight loss, but less than 10% of respondents used their phone to contact their doctors.

In a study by Miller et al. (2015), the three highest priorities for college students were: stress management linked to the mental health of young people; nutrition; and physical activity. In a qualitative study on the use of health and fitness apps among college students, Gowin et al. (2015) found that ease of app use is important, with cost of apps a barrier. Many participants said that their apps motivated them, coached them and sometimes even guilt-tripped or shamed them into performing their target behaviour. There was also resistance to sharing health and fitness activities on social media. There is a need for further research and understanding for health educators on use of health apps and social media for their health education programmes.

Considering the increasing use of health apps, particularly among young people, research in this area is at an early stage. Health apps tend to be directly available to consumers through, for example, Apple Store or Google Play. These apps tend to have no theoretical underpinning. Studies on the views and perspectives of users for behaviour change are also inadequate (Dennison et al. 2013). From Dennison et al.'s study, further investigation is important in resolving issues in app development such as focusing on long-term commitment to the use of health apps; the incorporation of behaviour change techniques such as goal setting and progress tracking; simplicity and low user burden; the provision of feedback on performance without generating adverse emotional reaction; and the context-sensing ability of health apps.

Implication for practice 2.1
Give three examples of how smartphone and health apps could help you in health promotion practice.

The new personal – wearables

Mobile phone apps are a logical development from phones and mobile phones. But there are newer usages and newer technologies. Consumer wearable devices promise to help individuals improve lifestyle behaviours such as physical activity, diet and sleep. The drivers for these are individuals' personal health behaviour and product/market development. In general, wearables such as activity trackers can help increase physical activity levels and are viewed positively (Maher et al. 2017). Smart wristbands serve a combination of utilitarian purpose, as well as an aesthetic function, with a gamified element. Research in the area of wristband usage is scarce, and people who use wristbands are expected to be more empowered to set personal health goals (Nelson et al. 2016). Nelson et al. found that wristbands influenced individual feelings of empowerment. This may be driven by multiple non-technical facets such as supportive communities and intrinsic motivation. Gamification and readability seem to be the strongest empowerment determinants in their study, though fashion may be important, with wristbands as fashion accessories.

Wearables are often used for measuring and monitoring the user's own health, turning the human body into a set of measurable data – the Quantified Self movement (personal data tracking to optimize health). Data help people to set goals and provide them with insights, and motivate them into changing their behaviour. Extrinsic rewards such as award badges reinforce behaviour.

Activity trackers can be more than just a tool to change behaviour. They can be incorporated into daily life, offering new social experiences, and new ways of boosting self-esteem and getting closer to our 'ideal selves': happiness in life. The intrinsic reward is about feeling good and healthy (Karapanos et al. 2016). If an activity is goal-orientated, performed for its beneficial impact – e.g. walking to get in shape – measurement may be helpful. However, Etkin (2016) argued that quantifying life in counting steps may decrease people's enjoyment of walking, as measurement even without external incentives could undermine our intrinsic motivation, decrease continued engagement and reduce enjoyment, making physical activity more like work.

Interestingly, Ledger (2014) found that 32 per cent of users stop wearing these devices after six months, and 50 per cent after a year. Key barriers were device breakage or loss, and technical difficulties with device software. Only a few users share their data on social media and special interest platforms such as Strava, a community platform that helps runners to connect and compete with each other (and with their own past achievement) via mobile and online apps (Maher et al. 2017). In a systematic review by Stephenson et al. (2017) on evaluations of the effectiveness of technology-enhanced solutions aimed at reducing sedentary behaviour, they found that interventions using computer, mobile and wearables can be effective in reducing such behaviour. However, the effect is more prominent in the short term and lessens over time, probably with decline of the novelty. There is a lack of follow-up measurement and evaluation on long-term reduction of sedentary behaviour.

There is evidence to support the validity of many wearables in accurately estimating physical activity and possibly promoting greater physical activity in the wearers (Farnell and Barkley 2017; Maher et al. 2017). Farnell and Barkley suggested that sharing and interacting of goals and behaviour with peers may explain an increase of physical activity among the wearers. Their pilot study on physical activity of women wearing Fitbit One showed that the group without the device (the control group) decreased in physical activity by more than 20 per cent, while the group with the device was largely unchanged (only decreased 0.5 to 2.4 per cent). They concluded that, while wearing a physical activity monitor didn't increase physical activity, it may help to maintain it.

Wearables can also be used to monitor health and wellbeing, aid rehabilitation, and relay adverse events such as falls, helping older people to live independently. Although there are limitations in the use of even research-grade wearables, they can help assess and monitor older people, providing information for independent living (Godfrey 2017). Piwek et al. (2016) found that wearables are more likely to be purchased by people who are already healthy and want to quantify progress. Manufacturers use persuasive techniques and social influences to engage users – e.g. gamification of activity with competition and challenges, publication of feedback on performance, using social influence principles or reinforcement, such as virtual rewards. An increasing number of people without medical training may seek medical advice, however, confused by the results from trackers. Practitioners and researchers need to work together to understand the impact of these advanced technologies (Melton et al. 2014; Piwek et al. 2016). Future developers also need to explore provision of feedback and ensure privacy protection.

Social media / social networking sites

The use of social media for health communication and to engage users in an interactive manner is increasingly common. The progression from Web 1.0 to Web 2.0 technology allows users to create, collaborate and share information – texts, photos and video – via the virtual environment. Social media are an extension of natural human social networking into online spaces (Brusse et al. 2014). We use software such as Facebook, Instagram, Twitter, etc., to communicate with each other remotely. The ability of social networking sites to generate direct communication, as well as two-way interactions between users, is particularly useful (Capurro et al. 2014). Web-based phones and smartphones can be used as behavioural intervention technologies (BITs) to reach large audiences cost-effectively, particularly the so-called 'hard to reach'. Capurro et al. cite the usage example of the Hispanic community in the United States (2014). Virtual-reality programmes can also help children with autism practise nonthreatening social interactions using graphics and customized avatars. Face-tracking technology can help build confidence and skills for real-world social applications (Gregoire 2014).

Online social media have become a novel setting for many health-related interventions, e.g. social marketing strategies, a consumer approach to selling social goods (discussed in more detail in chapter 4). Social media can have the reach of mass media, driven by small-scale social networking of ordinary people, and messages can 'go viral', radically magnifying reach and effect. By developing new relationships, and strengthening existing connections, social media can provide critical channels for the provision of health promotion (Ramanadhan et al. 2013; Thackeray et al. 2012). However, success or failure is difficult to predict. Health organizations have also been slow to develop digital health promotion interventions, as compared with commercial organizations. Among those using social media, many were still using it as one-way information provision, rather than as an interactive platform promoting engagement and participation (Ramanadhan et al. 2013; Thackeray et al. 2012). A survey from the Centre for Health Promotion, Women's and Children's Health Network (2012) found the vast majority of organizations don't use social media, and those who do only use Facebook and YouTube to engage clients and promote educational messages. Barriers include lack of resources, lack of guiding policy, lack of knowledge and skills, and lack of support from management.

Pagoto et al. (2014) investigate the use of Twitter for weight management. Their participants found greater support on Twitter than on Facebook from friends, and least from in-person family and friends. Possibly, people on Twitter share the same interest anonymously. You can 'unfollow' people much easier than on Facebook and in-person friends and family. There are benefits of social support and information sharing from the community without discomfort (Pagoto et al. 2014). Webb et al. (2010) found strongly theory-based interventions incorporating behaviour change techniques had more success. Tailored messages were highly effective – e.g. to send motivational messages, to challenge dysfunctional beliefs or to provide a cue for action. Communicative functions, such as giving advice or personal contact, can also support behaviour change. Sites that succeed tend to be highly dynamic and flexible, with regular content change to maintain audience interest.

There are health promotion challenges on social media, e.g. information overload, sustainability, effective tools for monitoring and evaluation as well as cost-effectiveness (Korda and Itani

2013). In a review on the use of social media for health promotion, Korda and Itani (2013) identified several key themes important in the development of social media for health promotion:

1 Target needs to be clearly identified, message needs to be appropriate for the audience. Health promotion model could be used to facilitate the process.
2 Keep up to date with current social media development.
3 Encourage engagement and participation.
4 Use different tools for multi-intervention strategies.
5 Need to be theory-based.
6 Need evaluation for monitoring effectiveness and activities-tracking.

Implication for practice 2.2
What would you need to think about if you needed to develop a social networking site to improve health service provision? Which type of social media would you choose and why? What kind of support and resources would you need for it to work effectively?

Use of digital technology among different groups of population and in different areas of health promotion

As already discussed, the Web 2.0 digital world is complex. Powerful stakeholders may be driven by profit and cost-effectiveness rather than evidence-based health outcomes. Governments, organizations and corporations focus on a medical model of health. Digital innovations may not achieve the health results they promise. There are equity and inequality issues through accessibility or usability. There are also challenging issues such as privacy and confidentiality. In the real world, some groups will benefit and some will be left behind. The following examples focus more on young people, since they are major users. Usage among other groups is also highlighted where research is available.

Young people

Twenty years ago, IT was not particularly the province of younger people. At best, families would have their own home-based, stand-alone consoles – it certainly was not a mobile and youth-centred phenomenon. Nowadays, children aged 8–11 are still quite similar in their usage to their peers of twenty years ago, mainly playing games on the computer, tablet or phones. The biggest change is among young people and young adults; those aged 12–17 are more interested in social interaction and social networking, with the internet now an important resource for young people. Around three-quarters of young people use the internet to seek out health information, and over half of 16- to 29-year-olds use their smartphone to access the internet. Roughly 90 per cent of 16- to 29-year-olds use the internet every day, and they spend more time online than any other group (Centre for Health Promotion, Women's and Children's Health Network 2012; Loss et al. 2014). Young people are digital residents (White and Le Cornu 2011) and naturally use the internet for information, as compared with older groups who are digital visitors. Similar to what we saw in the discussion on the use of wearables in the previous section, the extensive reach and functionality of social media among young people make online social networks promising platforms for health promotion topics such as physical activity (Cavallo et al. 2012).

In a study on the use of mobile apps by young people who live with HIV, by Saberi et al. (2016), participants frequently used their mobile phone to contact their medical provider. They used their devices to make appointments, for emailing, text messaging, but fewer used them for drug-related purposes, as compared with similar adults. The research concluded that the health app should focus on general health, not just HIV information. It should include a social network component, mechanisms to contact health service providers, a feature to track personal information, and a method to obtain HIV news and integrate clinical and behavioural components. However, issues of cost, privacy and confidentiality need further examination.

Rice et al. (2016), in an Australian study, found that many young Indigenous Australians use social media, reflecting their identity, culture and interactions with the wider world. This is despite economic, social, cultural and geographic factors – such as low attainment in education, education disengagement, child safety in experiencing abuse, and criminal justice system involvement – that can affect access. Indigenous young Australians used social media to strengthen identity, to feel a sense of power and control over their lives, and to maintain community and family connections. This could provide opportunities to improve education and health outcomes, in both urban and remote areas. Social media can also help improve inter-generational knowledge and relationships. Health promotion programmes using social media to promote active engagement can promote self-esteem, power and control, and resilience, increasing self-efficacy. However, Rice et al. (2016) also commented on negative aspects of social media, such as cyberbullying and abuse, cyber-racism and sexting, putting pressure on young people, and particularly damaging for people who are already vulnerable. Young people are exposed to unhealthy influences online, e.g. from food and drink advertising. Accessibility can also be an issue for some socially disadvantaged groups. There is also a contradiction in internet use for health promoters who at the same time are encouraging young people to reduce screen-time and increase physical activity. Rice et al. (2016) warned that health promotion programmes should not focus solely on changing individual behaviours. They should embrace wider approaches, including addressing the social determinants of health influencing individuals' health and wellbeing, as discussed by many authors, such as Lupton (2015c). Social determinants of health will be discussed in more depth in chapter 3.

Sexual health

Social networking sites also appear to be especially well suited to taboo topics such as sexual health, substance misuse and mental health. They have a broad potential reach for health communication, increasing the breadth and efficiency of health promotion messages, as well as for surveillance and research (Capurro et al. 2014). Positive sexual health programmes and applications, such as those helping women to keep track of ovulation and menstruation cycles and manage their fertility, are useful (Lupton 2015b). However, according to Gold et al. (2011), the use of social networking sites for sexual health promotion has been limited. Social networking sites tend to be US-based and for young people. They also primarily promote an organization, rather than positive sexual health messages. Lupton (2015b) agreed that most sexual health programmes are about problems associated with sexuality and sexual habits, rather than a wide range of positive sexual health issues.

A review by Bailey et al. (2015) on positive sexual health promotion among both young people and men having sex with men found that there are pockets of small local innovation but co-ordinated national programming is lacking in the UK as compared with other countries, particularly the USA. Most interventions also focus on risky behaviour and increased condom use, and few interventions are about sexual pleasure and positive relationships, or interventions which also look at alcohol and mental health (Bailey et al. 2015). They found a moderate effect on sexual health knowledge and a small effect on self-efficacy, but there was insufficient evidence on safer-sex intention or biological outcomes. Problems for widespread implementations include technical issues, clinical working patterns, lack of compulsory sex education in schools, reservations from teachers and parents, blocks on websites with online sexual content. The key factor for success is collaboration with stakeholders, particularly with young people themselves (as well as commercial and academic experts), for well-designed programmes in which quality and effectiveness are known and risks to young people minimized. Using an established social networking site (such as Facebook, Twitter) has the advantage that the audience is already present, rather than creating a customized platform which first has to attract users. However, the disadvantage of using general social media is that there is a lack of control of how health promotion activities are presented. Content also needs to be acceptable under site policy, and there are issues of ownership of the content. New technology provides tremendous opportunities for sexual health interventions among adolescents. More research focusing on behavioural outcomes is needed (Guse et al. 2012).

Estcourt et al. (2017) discussed the development of an eSexual health clinic for the management of *Chlamydia trachomatis* infection, from diagnosis to treatment, partner notification, health promotion and surveillance. *Chlamydia trachomatis* is the most commonly reported bacterial sexually transmitted infection (Public Health England 2016a). It mainly affects young people, the group that uses digital technology most. The results of their trial were positive, showing the safety and feasibility of the management of *Chlamydia* infection, with preliminary evidence of similar treatment outcomes to cases treated with traditional service. Estcourt et al. (2017) suggest that this type of eHealth initiative can also be applied to other infections and non-communicable diseases. However, they felt that the digital infrastructure and regulation of online medical care within the NHS is outdated. Data collection and surveillance of eHealth initiatives can be complicated. The efficacy, cost-effectiveness and public health impact need to be assessed.

Gold et al.'s (2012) Australian sexual health project FaceSpace, targeting young people and men who have sex with men, suggests that a multi-disciplinary team approach is important in developing health communication programmes, including health researchers, information technology experts, community organization experts. Ethical, legal and organizational concerns, such as privacy, intervention access, organizations' duty of care, and ownership, also need to be addressed. The cost of mass communication using the internet, where it can reach a large number of people, is cheap from a cost-per-head point of view; however, developing and maintaining the site and responding to the continuous flow of interactions from the public, as well as keeping the public engaged, require significant resources. The delivery of health interventions, and their reach and effect on the audience via internet space, are complex. In order for any intervention to achieve 'viral spread', the intervention must be well structured with a well-designed campaign and message to keep the audience engaged and to spread over cyberspace (Gold et al. 2012). Gold et al. found that the most popular sites are those with the most active online communities. There is a need to understand better how websites can be used for social engagement – e.g. the demographics of the users; how messages are spread; the impacts of activities on health knowledge, attitudes and behaviours; as well as the cost-effectiveness of interventions.

Positive sexual health resources for young people are clearly needed, and this is particularly true for young people in care, young parents, disabled young people, and lesbian and transgender young people. Young people have good access to digital technology; however, Mann and Bailey's (2016) review showed that websites and digital health education programmes are generally unregulated. Most digital interventions are for clinical use rather than health promotion. A literature review by Moorhead et al. (2013) showed a lack of good quality information about the use, benefits and limitations of social media in health communication.

The main benefits of social media identified were increased inter-actions, shared and tailored information, increased availability and accessibility of health information, peer/social/emotional support, public health surveillance and potential influencing of health policy. Limitations on the use of social media were mainly about quality concerns, lack of reliability, confidentiality and privacy. Social media, as a powerful tool, offer a new dimension to healthcare. However, information needs to be monitored for quality and reliability. User privacy and confidentiality also need to be maintained.

There is a lack of published literature on the use of social net-working sites promoting positive sexual health, possibly due to the rapidly emerging and changing use of social media. Lack of evidence has made it difficult for health professionals to search for published material, and to locate and learn from best practice (Gold et al. 2012; Moorhead et al. 2013). It is also difficult to define the term 'social media', as well as to measure health pro-motion activities in these media – unlike counting text-messaging. The fast-moving and changing field of digital technology also makes it difficult for research to be current. A better understand-ing of technology among professionals is needed, to understand how technology is being used. Further research is also needed on potential and effectiveness (Rice et al. 2016).

Digital stories

Another emerging way of using social media for health promotion is through digital storytelling. This can be useful for research and health promotion work. Digital video-making founded on partici-patory principles links to people's social context. Digital storytell-ing skills help engage communities effectively (O'Mara 2012). People are involved pre- and post-production through planning, script writing, design, and dissemination processes where messages can be posted online – e.g. commenting on the video on YouTube, using still images for those (such as refugees) lacking resources. A study by Fletcher and Mullett in Canada (2016) on the use of digital stories as a tool to promote health among young people found that the use of digital technology, building stories about healthy lifestyles with older people, can facilitate intergenerational interactions and community engagement. It is particularly useful in communities with a strong oral tradition and low literacy and e-literacy skills, since the internet tends to be text-dominated. Digital stories can complement traditional health promotion via drama, incorporating cultural and linguistic backgrounds into the story/narratives. The process of creating the story helps strengthen community relationships, allowing young people to create stories relevant to their own experience and communities, capturing their own voices. The process of creating stories helps people reflect on their experiences through the use of 'objects for reflection', a process of 'conscientization' – as described by Paulo Freire (1972) – encouraging dialogue and critical thinking, facilitating reflection and encouraging 'thinking about thinking', giving young people the opportunity to think deeply about a topic.

Mental health

Mental health problems among young people are well documented. In Australia, more than a quarter of young people aged 16–24 will experience mental illness in a 12 month period, with anxiety, substance abuse and mood disorders the most common. Three-quarters of the first episodes occur before age 25, but only 30% access professional help (Orlowski et al. 2015). Another survey by Lawrence et al. in 2015 showed that one in seven aged 4–17 in Australia were assessed as having mental disorders in the previous 12 months of the survey, with Attention Deficit Hyperactivity Disorder (ADHD) the most common (7.4%), followed by anxiety disorder (6.9%), depression (2.8%, more common in female and older adolescents) and conduct disorder (2.1%). However, 62.9% had received informal help or support, often from parents and friends, and only 3.6% (aged 13–17) reported using telephone counselling (though twice as many females as males) and 22.2% had used the internet – again females at double the rate of male users. The most common reasons for not seeking help related to stigma and poor mental health literacy. Online services could be useful to circumvent a range of barriers. Mental health promotion and prevention are needed to keep people mentally healthy in the first place. However, access to mental health online services by young people remains low (Lawrence et al. 2015; Ho et al. 2016; Sweeney et al. 2019).

Limited uptake and treatment adherence are important challenges for professionals (Orlowski et al. 2015). Horgan and Sweeney (2010) found university students' intentions to use online service are high. They valued privacy, accessibility, anonymity and confidentiality. Glasheen et al. (2015) also found 80–84 per cent of adolescents would consider using online counselling, if available in school. The involvement of an adult, providing support via telephone or email, can increase the adherence to treatment, but Mohr et al. (2013) found the improvement in health outcomes was not significant. Further improvement can be made if interventions have a greater therapeutic focus, more thoughtful use of multiple communication media, and longer contact. It is important to harness the power of technology, developing online platforms to deliver mental health services with great efficiency and scale (Hoise et al. 2014; Ho et al. 2016; Sweeney et al. 2019).

A Europe-wide survey carried out by the E-COMPARED consortium (Topooco et al. 2017) to assess the knowledge, acceptance and expectations of digital treatment for depression found that providers have a moderate knowledge of the potential benefits of digital interventions and consider cost-effectiveness a primary incentive for integrating digital technology into care services. The low feasibility of delivery within the present care system was a primary barrier. There was a high acceptance of blended treatments, with digital interventions offered in conjunction with standard face-to-face treatments. Digital treatment was more suitable for mild depression, though evidence shows internet-based treatments such as Deprexis were effective for adult depression even at a severe stage (Meyer et al. 2015; Semkovska and Ahern 2017). Internet-based treatment is sometimes considered impersonal, lacking face-to-face contact. Countries with better e-mental health, such as the Netherlands, Sweden and the UK, reported greater knowledge and more positive attitudes towards digital treatment than those with less developed e-mental health (such as France).

New technology has also been used for mental disorders such as eating disorders, schizophrenia, obsessive compulsive disorder, addictive behaviour and insomnia. According to the Sleep Council, nearly half of us are getting 6 hours or less of sleep, and four out of five complained of disturbed or inadequate sleep (Sleep Council 2011). Around 30 per cent of adults are reported to have insomnia, and 6–10 per cent meet the diagnostic criteria for insomnia disorder (Morin et al. 2009). Preliminary evidence shows that cognitive behavioural therapy delivered by an online automated support system and community forum appears effective in improving sleep and day-time functioning (Espie et al. 2012; Pillai et al. 2015).

Implication for practice 2.3
Think about health promotion in mental health and sexual health in general in your country – do you think digital technology can improve the service provision in this area? If yes, how can it improve services? If not, why not?

Mental health in low- and middle-income countries

Globally, there is poor access to mental healthcare, yet most people have access to a mobile phone (Kemp 2016). In many low-income countries in Africa, Central America and South Asia, more than 80% of the population are mobile phone subscribers, and internet access ranges from 27% in South Asia to 60% in South America. As much as 40% of global internet traffic comes from mobile devices – e.g. 66% in India, 70% in Indonesia, 82% in Nigeria and 75% in South Africa (Naslund et al. 2017). A World Bank report noted that the poorest households among the world's population are more likely to have access to mobile phones than to toilets or clean water (World Bank 2016). A narrative review by Naslund et al. (2017) shows a potential for online, text-messaging and phone-support interventions for low- and middle-income countries. Online tools such as education programmes have the potential to extend and develop the mental health workforce capacity and reach, connecting patients and community providers.

Mental health disorders such as depression are currently the major experience for people living with disability worldwide (Vos et al. 2015; Naslund et al. 2017). Low- and middle-income countries are disproportionately affected by this because of their underdeveloped healthcare systems (Patel et al. 2010). Globally, young people face challenges and barriers to healthcare, particularly in countries, such as those in Sub-Saharan Africa, with a high proportion of young people, with both poor youth health profiles and poor access to healthcare (Saraceno et al. 2007; Hampshire et al. 2015). Access to mobile networks is also useful for displaced populations and people in conflict zones, refugees and asylum-seekers. Technology could be the change driver in the improvement of care provision, and help to empower individuals, despite the potential risk of exposure to online harassment or negative influences. Evidence-based preventative interventions at population and community levels are needed (Patel et al. 2007, 2010; Petersen et al. 2016). However, implementation of mHealth initiatives and evidence of their effects are limited, needing significant investment (Bloomfield et al. 2014; Chib et al. 2014; Hampshire et al. 2015). More attention to politics, leadership, planning, advocacy and participation, as well as resources, are also necessary (Saraceno et al. 2007; Naslund et al. 2017).

Young people use their mobile phones creatively and strategically. In low- and middle-income countries such as Ghana, Malawi and South Africa, young people have themselves developed mHealth informally, e.g. calling for help, searching for health information and getting advice. This seems to support a neoliberal view of empowerment, choice and responsibility. However, it shifts responsibility for healthcare provision from the state to young people themselves. Access to health services is not a level playing field, with serious consequences (e.g. the risk of navigating a potential minefield of misinformation). The lack of access to technology, coupled with poor health service provision, is particularly intense in impoverished rural areas. There is a need for diverse initiatives, such as the use of solar chargers to compensate for unreliable supplies of electricity, a more proactive role for governments in healthcare provision, and better education programmes for young people in building digital capital. There is also a need to accelerate investment in universal health coverage and youth-friendly services, where active participation from young people themselves would be important (Hampshire et al. 2015).

Gamification – Active Video Games (AVGs)

Video games were originally developed as entertainment, but they have long been used for education purposes. Now they have become useful for health. 'Gamification' is a term used to describe the use of game design in a non-game context, aimed at motivating and improving user experience and engagement, encouraging people to take their own responsibility for their health and promoting sustained behaviour change for good health (Cross et al. 2017). Computer and video games can be valuable for children in hospital, both for education and for entertainment. Video gaming has been a multi-billion-dollar industry in the USA. Most research focuses on the harm from video gaming, e.g. violence, inactivity, obesity, risk-taking behaviours and poor school performance. However, in recent years, there has been an increase in active video games (AVGs) aiming to increase physical activity and reduce obesity (Primack et al. 2012).

Sedentary lifestyle and inactivity are contributing factors for obesity in children. One in five school children is overweight (Centers for Disease Control and Prevention (CDC) 2017). Being overweight has implications for physical and mental health. It increases the risk of Type 2 diabetes, asthma, cardiovascular disease and premature death. Obesity also subjects children to bullying, social isolation, depression and low self-esteem, as well as missing school days. Obesity is now a global epidemic, including in countries where undernutrition is common. According to the WHO (2017b), 155 million children were affected by stunting in 2016, 52 million children were wasting, while 41 million were overweight. Of child deaths worldwide, 20 per cent are related to malnutrition. Paradoxically, low-birthweight babies and stunting are both risk factors for children becoming overweight. The 'Double burden' of malnutrition is a term given to the presence of both obesity and underweight in the same population, community or family.

Exercise is a critical component in health maintenance and disease prevention (Albu et al. 2015). Playing video games is popular among adolescents. Video gaming, an 'inactivity' activity seen as not to be encouraged, however, can have huge benefits for children with chronic conditions such as diabetes, asthma, poor mental health, etc. Well-produced video games have been used for behaviour changes, e.g. in areas of physical activity (Lister et al. 2014) and in patients with cancer, pain, stroke, obesity and mental disorder (Concepcion 2017; Fernández-Aranda et al. 2012). Assistive technology treatments using interactive video game therapy can promote health. They can also be used to distract people from pain, and for education purposes and health-related activities such as training of healthcare professionals.

Video gaming as exercise programming can also be highly accessible, highly motivating, with wide market penetration (Sony, Nintendo, Microsoft – PlayStation Move, Wii, Xbox Kinect). Exercise games (exergames) such as BringItOn promote proper exercise techniques with on-screen feedback, acting as a personal trainer with rewards. Participants can exercise in the comfort of their home. This kind of video-based gaming can help health promotion and address the motivation challenge by being fun and entertaining (Albu et al. 2015). It promotes exercise and calorie burning through repeated motions based on intrinsic motivation where one engages in an activity for enjoyment (Simons et al. 2014). However, a concern about console exergames is that they might replace traditional forms of outdoor exercise, such as cycling, which require greater energy expenditure. But exergames coupled with GPS with a mobile device (GPS exergames) – such as MovesCount App Zone, Suunto's App Designer – can be played outdoors in different locations. Exergames can also have problems – e.g., in game-player safety, and adjusting to the player's physical ability (Boulos and Yang 2013). Further research is needed to assess the trade-off inherent in the use of video games instead of other modalities (Primack et al. 2012).

For many reasons (e.g. physical barriers, poor disabled access, lack of supportive personnel or financial support), obesity prevalence and physical inactivity are higher among disabled young people, compared with their non-disabled counterparts. Exergames can be seen as a 'gateway experience' to promote health for this group. A conceptual model of active gaming developed by the Rehabilitation Engineering Research Centre on Interactive Exercise Technologies and Exercise Physiology for people with disabilities (RERC RecTech), showing the accessibility barriers and the contextual factors involving the 'person' and the 'environment', can be used to explain the increased health benefit of AVGs. Games that can adapt to the player's ability level could expand the benefit of AVGs (Rowland et al. 2016). In another study by Hsieh et al. (2016) on video games for children with developmental delay, the authors found that short-term interactive video game play in conjunction with traditional therapies improved physical health. However, there was no significant improvement of psychological health, functional performance or family impact. Video games may have the potential for health improvement in a wide variety of areas for a wide variety of sociodemographic groups. However, most studies conducted have been of poor quality with relatively brief follow-up periods. There is also a need to understand the theory underpinning exergames, such as motivation and social cognitive theory (Boulos and Yang 2013). Further research is also needed to demonstrate effectiveness (Primack et al. 2012).

Gamification – serious game

Children learn through play. Using games for educational purposes is a well-established and well-recognized way for teaching and promoting active learning – for example, in traditional subjects such as maths, sciences, geography and reading. 'Serious gaming' includes electronic games with a therapeutic purpose that are commonly used for health-related education, for example about healthy eating, drug misuse and sensitive topics such as sex education (Bowen et al. 2014). Combating and preventing violence against women and girls is an important area where schools and teachers have a role to play (Council of Europe 2011). Although this is not a statutory topic in formal school education in UK, many schools do include this in their Personal, Social and Health Education curriculum. 'Green Acres High' was a game developed to raise awareness among adolescents of date-violence, and to promote healthy relationships. Through a qualitative study, Bowen et al. (2014) found that the learning experience via a digital medium was clearly positive. The game was pedagogically underpinned by experiential learning. Students learn through the interactive element of the game, an autonomous and student-centred learning where they have to make choices and decisions, developing their problem-solving skills. The participants also felt motivated to learn. It was suggested that the use of digital technology can be included alongside traditional learning. This is a small preliminary study and the results were inconclusive. It appears that negative experiences were due to technical deficiencies, lack of IT capacity and IT support, or the IT infrastructure of the school, rather than the deficiency of serious gaming itself. Further study is recommended.

Serious games complement traditional treatments in the mental health setting, often more enjoyably and acceptably for both therapists and patients (Horne-Moyer et al. 2014). With present difficulties in accessing healthcare services, modern technology and electronic games can be interesting, readily available and delivered efficiently. Horne-Moyer et al. (2014) reviewed both serious games and off-the-shelf games for leisure purposes, such as Xbox games, used as therapeutic tools. Both types of games have been used in health promotion to improve the physical and psychosocial functioning of patients. While electronic games for psychotherapy are designed specifically for the needs of the patients, other electronic games with gross motor interface such as Xbox Kinect can provide physical challenges, improving physical fitness, and sedentary games help improve knowledge and healthy behaviour. Electronic games can also be used in areas such as stress management, confidence building, and socialization. In their review, electronic methods have shown to be equivalent in efficacy for a range of medical and mental health issues, among groups, individuals, and for self-guided treatment. Fernández-Aranda et al. (2012), in another European multi-centre project, PlayMancer, also looked at a serious game which uses biofeedback to help patients learn relaxation skills, and improve self-control and emotional regulation strategies. Initial results were positive in enhancing the long-term effectiveness of traditional therapies.

Electronic methods can be more acceptable, enjoyable and engaging than traditional therapies. Electronic games for healthcare purposes need to be selected based on their appeal to users and their potential for meeting therapeutic needs. Parents also need to be educated on risks and protective factors – e.g. playing with children to monitor their play for duration and content. Children should be encouraged to play with friends rather than using online services, particularly if socialization and social skills are important therapeutic goals. Studies suggest that computer-assisted therapies can offer treatments that are equally as effective as, and require less time and less therapist involvement than, traditional models of care. They can also provide better access for people in rural or underserved areas. Online services can be incorporated in a professional and engaging manner (Horne-Moyer et al. 2014). However, cost-effectiveness is unclear. More evidence and rigorous evaluations are needed on their effective use for cognitive enhancement in mental health (Fernández-Aranda et al. 2012; Barrett and Gershkovich 2013; Bisoglio et al. 2014). The support and training of therapists is important, e.g. how treatments are determined and issues regarding consent, confidentiality, ethics, as well as inequality issues. A review by Ricciardi and De Paolis (2014) found that serious gaming can improve learning and skill development of healthcare professionals. Virtual reality, such as traditional simulators with computer technology, is useful – e.g. in first-aid training – particularly when continuous professional development is important. However, the use of serious games is not widespread.

Reflection 2.2

Many people are addicted to playing games – children and adults alike. Thinking about the principles and value of health promotion, what is your view on using games as a vehicle for health promotion?

Chronic ill-health management / telehealth and telecare

Telehealth is the remote exchange of data between an individual and healthcare professionals. It can be particularly useful in managing existing long-term conditions such as chronic obstructive pulmonary disease (COPD), diabetes or heart failure. It often includes remote transmission of clinical signs, and video or email consultations (Honeyman et al. 2016). Telecare is the remote monitoring of an individual's condition or lifestyle in their home environment. It aims to manage risk in an Independent Living setting. Sensors can now monitor falls or bed occupancy, making home healthcare viable. The number of people today aged 60-plus has doubled since 1980. Within the next five years, adults over 65 will outnumber children under 5 and, by 2050, will outnumber children under 14. Even in low-income countries, most people die from non-communicable diseases. The number of people living with disability is also increasing – e.g., people with dementia (WHO 2012). Each year, millions of people die of preventable illness such as coronary heart diseases (CHD), COPD, HIV, lung cancer or diabetes (WHO 2011b).

There are three main applications in the use of technology for patient engagement in complex health conditions. They are: self-care advice and routine transactions; support in self-management of long-term conditions; and remote monitoring to help patients to be cared for at home (Coulter and Mearns 2016). Telehealth and telecare have been used since the early 2000s, particularly in the care of long-term conditions. They can play a role in empowering and supporting patients and their carers. Evidence bases and cost-effectiveness are, however, not conclusive (Goodwin 2012). In England, the government is committed to the use of technology, as seen in the *NHS Five Year Forward View* document (National Health Service 2014, 2017). Currently, in the UK, only a few NHS Trusts use telehealth and telecare (Honeyman et al. 2016). The concern is that most of these technologies only require passive involvement. Control remains with health professionals who monitor results and make decisions. It is good that patients don't need to travel to clinics, but it may not enhance their self-management capability, undermining their sense of self-efficacy, encouraging them to depend on machines without increasing their confidence in their own self-care efforts (Sanders et al. 2012). Patients and carers need to be actively involved to be truly empowered (Coulter and Mearns 2016).

In diabetes management, patient involvement is important, particularly in self-management and shared decision making (Weymann et al. 2014). The internet provides health information for people with diabetes to learn and manage their condition at their own pace, becoming the expert in their own care. A study of German and English diabetes website quality by Weymann et al. (2014) showed most websites provide basic information necessary for decision making, but only a few have specific information for shared decision making between patient and professional. Most websites do not provide sufficient information to support patients in medical decision making. Websites with a quality code have better formal quality criteria scores. No website said that patients were involved in website development. There is a highly significant correlation between usability of the website and website traffic, as well as a significant correlation between formal quality and website traffic, indicating that the design and appearance of websites is important for web users in assessing website credibility.

The development of digital technology and the use of telehealth and telecare in managing chronic health conditions is a global phenomenon. An example from one of the author's students in South Africa shows digital technologies used since March 2018 in delivering medication for patients with chronic illnesses. This system has reduced the burden on clinic facilities, reduced patient waiting time and allowed patients to access their medication closer to their homes. It was also helpful to non-clinical staff. An evaluation is yet to be completed, 12 months after the programme started (Mpongwana 2018, unpublished).

There is a concern that increased technology use is technologically driven. Technology can offer disabled or frail older people a degree of empowerment – the technology is assistive. However, some would argue that one may become dependent on technology (Milligan et al. 2011), or the design may be ill thought-through. From a study by Milligan et al. (2011), it was found that surveillance and monitoring tools can be seen as invading people's privacy in their own home, changing people's front room into an institution with the installation of technology; the sense of being watched by someone around the clock can be unnerving, 'warehousing' people in their own home. Technology can't replace human contact. Care can become technocratic, a 'medicalized' approach – people can be isolated in their own home. It may address the physical needs of older people (as defined by a professional), but not necessarily mental health needs or social and affective needs. It also may not help people with memory loss, as in dementia, or people with hearing or sight impairment. Technology must be used as an aid for care, rather than a solution to replace personal care. Technology design needs to involve the people themselves to determine what is useful for them, based on their needs.

Reflection 2.3

Is telecare/telehealth well developed/used in your area/country of practice? How can it be developed further? What infrastructure, support and resources need to be in place?

Summary conclusion

Digital technology has been a fast-developing industry in the last twenty years, with many possibilities – e.g. the increased design of wearables, social networking sites, the use of digital stories. Online services are particularly useful for sensitive issues such as mental health and sexual health. The potential risks of sharing information online, data safety and security, also need to be looked at (Bloomfield et al. 2014; Naslund et al. 2017). We need to be critical when citing evidence to support practice. Many reviews have found that studies on the use of digital technologies were weak. Rigorous research is needed to assess its feasibility, acceptability and effectiveness.

Digital technologies may be able to contribute to the efficient and effective running of health services, and to support communities and individuals in promoting and maintaining health. There is a complex interaction between digital technology, societal factors and health. There is also a complex interplay between digital innovation, the globalized marketplace and our understanding of health. We need to think beyond one-way, top-down information transfer. It is about relationships and inter-relationships. The flows and pressures from technological developments, globalization and consumerist power (all within a dominant neoliberal system) led to the phenomenon of Big Data. People can become mesmerized by technological innovation, their lives reduced to a set of measurements and the pathological treatment of illness. We need to become health-focused, not innovation-focused or sickness-focused. There is a need to develop a more critical vision of what technology can do for us and how it can make a difference.

This review provides a lot of details on the applications of digital technology in practice. There are some areas that we will need to look at in more depth in the rest of this book, in order fully to understand its implications:

- Digital technology offers a lot of opportunities for health promotion. However, there is a danger that we may get lost in the commercialization of innovation. We need to be critical about its claims and our belief in its cost-effectiveness. There is a need to work with technology users, with a sound theoretical underpinning and resourced provision.
- Technology can be empowering or disempowering. Self-management of health and taking responsibility for your own health can be framed as 'empowerment' while simply shifting responsibility of healthcare provision from the government to the individual. It is also about the digital divide – between those who have access and know how to use technologies, and those without access, or who don't have the skills in using technology.
- Behaviour can become pathological and interventions medicalized, ignoring what health actually means and how it can be

influenced. In many ways, the literature on digital innovation in health has not caught up with the literature on health promotion. There is a need to understand the principles and value of health promotion actions.

- The development of digital technology provides a lot of strength and opportunities, but also weaknesses and threats. We need to be aware of power relationships in the digital world and gain better understanding of the issues of choices, power and empowerment. They can cause problems for those who use the technologies – such as data security – but also be problematic to those left behind.

3

The Alignment of Digital Health Promotion to Health Promotion Principles and Values

Key points

- To discuss the use of digital technologies in health communication.
- To explore what is meant by 'health' and how health can be promoted digitally, relating to the principles and values of health promotion.
- To consider the determinants of health and underpinning theory for health promotion in relation to digital health promotion.
- To discuss power, choice and control, principles of empowerment and participation in digital health.
- To consider the use of digital platforms as a virtual setting for health promotion.
- To discuss health promotion ethics relating to digital health interventions.

Introduction

Health is a resource for everyday life (WHO 1986). Modern ill health includes issues such as obesity, smoking, drinking, and complications such as coronary heart disease, hypertension, stroke, diabetes, often caused by unhealthy lifestyles. Good health depends on many social determinants, for example education, employment, housing, transport (WHO 2010). Health promotion is a social movement (Dixey 2013), and health is a political choice (WHO 2016). Based on the Social Model of Health, healthy living cannot simply be achieved top-down (WHO 2016). Promoting health is a shared responsibility requiring global collective actions, seeking to address all determinants of health and removing barriers to empowerment. Considering the concept of Salutogenesis, we can learn to cope with life-stresses with a high sense of coherence, moving towards optimal wellbeing (Antonovsky 1996). Health promotion is about empowering and enabling people to make healthy choices in a health-supporting environment. Healthy public health and social policy are essential in providing that health-supporting environment for individuals and communities to make healthy choices and maintain a high sense of coherence, increasing citizens' control of their own health.

Empowerment approaches helping to build social capital and promote asset-based health improvement figured prominently in the 2016 WHO Global Health Promotion conference. The use of digital technology for health communication has the potential to promote individual and community empowerment, advocating for better health. In public health, media space and virtual reality have recently become a new 'setting' (a communicative social venue) for health promotion (Gold et al. 2012; Loss et al. 2014). However, it also has a potential risk of disempowering some population groups, e.g. socially and economically disadvantaged communities, disabled people, and a range of resource-poor population groups (Lupton 2015c; Cross et al. 2017).

This chapter will look at the use of digital technologies in relation to the principles, values and practice of health promotion as discussed in the Ottawa Charter (WHO 1986), and the neglect of social, cultural, economic and environmental determinants of health; and discuss how a Salutogenic approach to positive health (Becker et al. 2010) might be enhanced through the use of digital technologies. It will assess how digital technology might be able to offer, in alignment with health promotion principles and values, a way to assess critically the implications of digital technologies in health promotion practice and health promotion goals as described by the WHO (2016): 'promoting health, promoting sustainable development: Health for all and all for Health'.

Health communication and digital technology

As noted in chapter 2, digital technologies are widely used in healthcare. According to Whiting and Williams (2013), 88 per cent of web users use social media for social interaction and 80 per cent for information-seeking. Through digital technology, health promotion messages can be sent to individuals interpersonally as well as to mass audiences. They can be personalized and targeted for an individual according to their needs, e.g. via text messaging. With accelerometers and GPS systems, individuals can be located spatially, and assessed and monitored – e.g., in chronic health conditions where patients can contact their health professionals directly from their home. With narrowcasting and audience segmentation, tailored messages can be used to target certain user groups. Health messages can also be embedded into entertainment programmes such as dramas. Media such as blogs, Twitter, podcasts, etc., can also be used as communication tools to update followers, although tweets can be a cause for misunderstanding and abuse of health information (Scanfeld et al. 2010). Conversation over the internet is interactive and relational. The social and cultural context is important (Kreuter and McClure 2004). However, as with much mass media communication, conversation over the net can be impersonal. Much non-verbal communication is missing, even with synchronized discussion. Feedback can also be delayed if the communication is asynchronous. The advantage of internet communication is its mass access at population level. However, there is no control on who the target audience is, and engagement is also difficult to measure.

Communication using Web 1.0 technology resembles one-way communication where communication is top-down, linear, a monologue without feedback, as described by Lasswell's classic communication model (1948), or the Shannon–Weaver model (1949) with the interference of 'noise' in the external environment or internal life experience background. This 'arrow' approach of information transfer, as described by Clampitt (2001), has a persuasive intent. It is like giving a lecture in a large lecture theatre. The power of the expert over passive people ignores the social, cultural, environmental and structural barriers or the lived experience of the information receivers (McQuail and Windahl 1993).

Communication using Web 2.0 technology resembles two-way information exchange, in which feedback is an important element (Cross et al. 2017), as seen in Osgood and Schramm's (Schramm 1954) circular model of communication. Communication is cyclical. Clampitt described this as the 'circuit' approach, where both information senders and receivers act as coders and decoders, simultaneously interpreting information as they receive it. There is a dialogue and interaction, stimulating critical thinking and a bottom-up information processing. This dialogical importance of communication implies an equal relationship, and can lead to empowering change among individuals as well as societally (McQuail and Windahl 1993; Cross et al. 2017).

In health promotion, feedback is important for checking accuracy and evaluating effectiveness of the intended message, as seen in Hubley (2004) and Green et al.'s (2015) health communication model demonstrating how a health message can be passed forward and backward via a communication channel. There is a social relationship, context-orientated, taking into account the agency of the information recipients. Health information is not just received, but thought about and acted upon. However, the challenge of health promotion is in the motivation of the information receivers to make change upon receipt of information (Cross et al. 2017). Health promotion has traditionally been a low-tech area of public health, as compared with acute medicine. Even Web 1.0 technology, although a static technology, can be very valuable in public information provision. The interactivity of Web 2.0, the social web with the characteristics of collaboration and participation, has in turn increased personal empowerment and social change, allowing a two-way communication and real-time feedback, adding value to user engagement (Hanson et al. 2008; Lupton 2012).

In health communication on the internet, we can see that the audience is active. Linking this to the 'uses and gratifications' theory, audiences actively seek information or participate on the net. People choose media messages that suit their own needs and interests, align with their own beliefs and values – e.g., for information, for relaxation. They interact with and interpret the messages selectively, using the media to gratify their desires and satisfy their prejudices (McQuail 2010; Green et al. 2015). Hence, they may not interpret the messages as was intended by the message producer. This also demonstrates the limitations of mass media penetration, as shown by the 'aerosol spray' theory in which some messages hit the target and most drift away with little effective penetration, and the limitations of the 'hypodermic' theory, in which a direct influence on an individual occurs, like an injection (Green et al. 2015; Cross et al. 2017). Web 2.0 users are 'prosumers'. They produce and consume digital content at the same time, producing user-generated content (Ritzer et al. 2012). Participation and co-production of content are at the centre of communication strategies, changing broadcasting to conversation. The characteristics of social media can align well with the Ottawa Charter, e.g. strengthening community actions, developing personal skills and creating supportive environments (Norman 2012). It can also contribute to the process of developing healthy public policies and reorientation of health services.

Determinants of health and upstream health promotion

Building on the Lalonde report in 1974 (Lalonde 1974), the Declaration on Primary Healthcare at Alma-Ata in 1978 (WHO 1978), the Global Strategy for Health for All by year 2000 (WHO 1981), and many debates within the new public health movement around the world, the Ottawa Charter was the result of the first international conference on health promotion in 1986. Health is a resource, created and lived by people within the settings of their everyday life. Health promotion is about enabling people to increase control over and improve their own health (WHO 1986). The prerequisites for health include peace, shelter, education, food, income, a stable ecosystem, sustainable resources, social justice and equity. Therefore, it involves a wide range of enabling social, economic and environmental conditions. The action areas include building healthy public policies, creating supportive environments, strengthening community actions, developing personal skills and reorienting health services. These five action areas and the three strategies of health promotion – enable, mediate and advocate – encapsulate health promotion.

The United Nations (UN) announced their commitment to Agenda 2030 ensuring a safer, fairer and healthier world by 2030, via the seventeen Sustainable Development Goals (SDGs) (UN 2015). At the health promotion conference in Shanghai (WHO

2016), the WHO reaffirmed the relevance of the Ottawa Charter, and that this can only be achieved through the SDGs. It emphasized the need for universal health coverage and reducing health inequities for people of all ages, leaving no one behind. As seen through a series of WHO global health promotion conferences over the years (WHO 1986, 1988, 1991, 1997, 2000, 2005b, 2009, 2013, 2016), healthy public policies and addressing inequality and inequity in health and society are two main discussions throughout all such conferences. Health promotion involves the participation and collaboration of the whole population and all organizations – local, national and international. Intersectoral action is needed and all stakeholders have a role in addressing social determinants of health and building capacity in health promotion. The central element is that health is a fundamental right.

The social determinants of health have been discussed for many years. The well-known Dahlgren and Whitehead (1991) diagram successfully showed the different layers of influences on a person's health, from their genetics, age and gender to their individual lifestyle, their social and community networks, their living and working conditions, and the wider economic, cultural and environmental conditions. There is a more than forty-year difference in life expectancy between countries, and there are dramatic social gradients in health within countries. Progress can be made towards closing this gap by improving the conditions in which people are born, grow, live, work and age, for example in dealing with inequity in power, money and resources (Commission on Social Determinants of Health (CSDH) 2008). Upstream health promotion is about improving these social, environmental and economic determinants in the upstream, creating an enabling and supportive environment, so that people won't fall into the stream in the first place, rather than having to be rescued when they are drowning downstream. In the UK, a review of health inequalities in England recommended six domains for action to improve health – (i) give every child the best start in life; (ii) improve education and lifelong learning; (iii) create fair employment and jobs; (iv) ensure a minimum income for a healthy standard of living; (v) build healthy and sustainable communities; and (vi) apply a social determinants approach to prevention (Marmot 2010). As can be seen, for digital health promotion to work, it needs to be able to foster collaborative, participatory upstream working strategies.

Does digital health align with health promotion principles and values?

The normative ideal of health promotion is about equity, equality and social justice. Health promotion is therefore a value-based, political and ethical activity at individual, community and population levels. There is a clear narrative about tackling the social determinants of health. However, the top-down education approach, dominant before the Ottawa Charter, still dominates, as does the pathological medical model of health. Despite the health promotion movement's efforts through the 1980s and 1990s, 'information provision' and 'advice giving' remain the healthy-living norm. As discussed in chapter 2, digital health promotion focuses on a behaviour- and lifestyle-change approach. This behaviour-change approach, together with the traditional education and medical approach, distances health promotion practice from its normative ideal.

Health education has been key to health promotion. Education based on dialogue stimulates critical thinking, a process of consciousness-raising, rather than 'banking' knowledge into an empty vessel (Freire 1973). Through education, the learners' world is 'decoded'. Education is the catalyst for personal and social change. It is about raising people's consciousness of health issues, to be able to make choices and eventually create pressure for healthy public policies, transforming society (Naidoo and Wills 2009). Freire highlights the social dimension of the education process and challenges individualistic perspectives. Aligned to Dewey's (1916) and Freire's (1973) thinking, Green et al. (2015) asserted that effective 'critical health education' that involves 'critical thinking' facilitates the development of the individual's cognitive capabilities, improving their decision-making skills and bringing about changes free from coercion. According to Mezirow's transformative learning (1997, 2003), one has to be willing to learn and to participate. This involves critical thinking and critical reflection. Facing challenging perspectives, one could step over into another realm of understanding – cross the 'threshold', a shift of consciousness as discussed by Meyer et al. in the threshold concept (2010).

Health literacy can provide a way to empower individuals and communities. It can support greater autonomy and personal empowerment, equipping people to overcome structural barriers to health (Nutbeam 2000). Critical health education and healthy public policies are the two main elements in bringing about health in Green et al.'s empowerment model of health promotion (2015). An oppressive environment can have dramatic effects on an individual's health and their capacity to make choices (Green et al. 2015). The empowering function of education strengthens the individual's capacity in decision making for health as well as contributing to the development of healthy public policies. It is essential for a health-promoting and health-enabling environment.

The interactiveness of Web 2.0 technology with two-way communication can provide a dialogical approach to health communication. However, it is not always easy for someone to be able to learn, to participate, to think and reflect critically in an ever-changing virtual environment. Not only do the learners need to engage in the learning process actively, the health promoters and web developers also need to facilitate learning to enable transformation to occur. It can also be difficult to practise health promotion in keeping with the normative ideals, particularly when there are debates on what being healthy actually means. Considering the above discussion on what health promotion is about, digital health promotion as discussed in chapter 2 focuses on individualistic behaviour and lifestyle changes, and is far from meeting the normative ideal of health promotion. Concepts such as equity, equality, justice, empowerment and participation are open to interpretation. This involves value judgements and ethical debates. For example, how do we square the promotion of citizens' autonomy regarding their health with expecting health promotion professionals to encourage people, sometimes persuasively, to pursue health-related goals? How can we use technology in ways that help to address social justice, health equity and health inequality? How we use technology depends on our beliefs, which translates to our practice. In order to contextualize how digital health can be used in health promotion practice, it is also important to recognize the different understandings of health.

Health and health promotion

The dominant definition of health is about the absence of disease, a scientific, western biomedical model – a negative view of health.

The WHO's definition of health as a state of complete physical, mental and social wellbeing, not merely the absence of disease or infirmity, is holistic; it does include positive aspects (WHO 1946). However, it still focuses on the absence of disease. In the case of public health medicine, health is, again, viewed through the lens of sickness; measuring health with indicators such as mortality, morbidity, prevalence, incidence, risk factors, life expectancy, etc. We can see this in digital health promotion – e.g. health apps, wearables – as well as in chronic ill-health management, where we constantly quantify ourselves, measuring and tracking our bodily functions and comparing ourselves with 'normal parameters' and with others, and set goals and targets towards these parameters.

Given the risk of developing chronic health conditions in the present day, Huber et al. (2011) argue that many of us would be classified as unhealthy. They proposed that the formulation of health should be the ability to adapt and to self-manage. From lay perspectives, health can mean different things to different people. For example, older people tend to think of health as wholeness, inner strength, ability to cope (Williams 1983), and younger people tend to define health from a fitness point of view. People from the middle classes tend to link health to enjoying life, being fit and active, whereas lower social-economic groups tend to define health based on their ability to function. A later and more comprehensive definition from WHO (1984) stated that health is 'the extent to which an individual or group is able, on the one hand, to realize aspirations and satisfy needs, and on the other hand, to change or cope with the environment. Health is therefore seen as a resource for everyday life, not the object of living.' This view is more positive, emphasizing social and personal resources and physical capabilities, an asset-based definition (WHO 1986). However, the concept of health as a resource has not really been explored in depth, despite frequent references to it (Huber et al. 2011).

Although promoting health as a resource could foster individuals' investment in health, Williamson and Carr (2009) note that this does not fully represent laypeople's experiences and understandings of health. We live in a pluralistic/multi-cultural/multi-racial society, and it is important to understand a person's health in different social contexts. In contrast to the medical model of health emphasizing individuals' responsibilities for health, the social model of health takes a holistic view. Health is not governed by the structure and function of the body, but by the social world in which we live. Ill health is caused by social factors, social conditions, and medicine itself is part of the social world. With the recognition of the social determinants of health, the social model of health has gained more acceptance in the health promotion field as a holistic, multi-dimensional concept, emphasizing social responsibility for health (Dixey 2013). Reflecting on the discussion in chapter 2, does the use of digital technology in health echo the 'upstream' health promotion ideals? How can we use digital technology in a social model of health context to address our understanding of health, which is influenced by many social determinants?

For many years, disease-orientated health education and awareness-raising emphasized lifestyle changes and behaviour approaches to promote health. The success of this approach is unclear, and it has lacked theoretical underpinning in health promotion interventions. Yet the development and the use of digital technology in health promotion continue to emphasize this approach. From a commentary by Watt (2002) on reviewing oral health education, he found that psychological theory was used as the theoretical framework even though it had been highlighted that there are shortcomings in psychological concepts and knowledge–attitude–behaviour models. Alternative theories which acknowledge wider determinants of health are needed. The three theories cited in his paper were:

- Life course perspective – biological risk interacts with economic, social and psychological factors in the development of chronic illness through the whole life course. An individual's disease status is a marker of their past social position (e.g. poor child health links to adult chronic health condition; the impact of unemployment on later health and life).
- Salutogenesis – stressors are standard features in life. Individuals and communities with a strong sense of coherence are better equipped to deal with these stressors and maintain good health. Identifying and modifying the social and structural environment can move the population towards health on the health–disease continuum.

- Social capital – this is a feature of social organization, such as participation, trust, how safe people feel. The better the social support, social network, social cohesion, the better the health. Growing gaps between rich and poor affect social organization and have implications for public health.

Health promotion is multi-disciplinary, but many analysts are concerned that there is still no theoretical basis for health promotion practice and the principles of the Ottawa Charter (Antonovsky 1996; Eriksson and Lindstrom 2008). Eriksson and Lindstrom noted that this causes problems for the health promotion movement, particularly as the current societal paradigm is dominated by the traditional pathogenic medical model of health. For laypeople and health professionals alike, health is still about sickness, and getting better relies on behaviour change and individual responsibility, as seen in many digital health promotion interventions. Watt (2002) and Eriksson and Lindstrom (2008) have suggested that the Salutogenic approach could offer a framework for health promoters in their research and practice. It harmonizes well with the essence of the Ottawa Charter. It reflects the diversity of health promotion practice, which is not just about individual behaviour, but about society and its organization. In fact, community development and healthy public policies leading to a healthy society are central to the Charter.

The focus of health promotion work is clear. It is about health, not disease. According to Antonovsky (1996), we cannot simply be labelled healthy or diseased, we are all located somewhere along the health–disease continuum. Contrary to the pathogenic model, the Salutogenic approach asserts that humans are flawed and susceptible to diseases and injury; we need to be active to stay healthy. Health promotion is about identifying factors helping us to move along the continuum. Thus, rather than eradicate certain stressors, we adapt, develop positive approaches to enhance our wellbeing. The sense of coherence in the Salutogenic theory is based on three dimensions – *Comprehensibility*, whereby you can make sense of the things around you; *Manageability*, where you believe you have the resources necessary to take care of things, that things are manageable and within your control; and *Meaningfulness*, where life makes sense emotionally and is worth living. As health promotion is about enabling and empowering, working towards positive health with the core values of equity, participation and empowerment, Eriksson and Lindstrom (2008) argue that these are also the central elements in the Salutogenic concept. Web 2.0 digital technology has much to offer in health promotion, as seen in tailored messaging and the use of social networking sites in the provision of support in a virtual community, promoting both individual and community empowerment.

Upstream health promotion is about keeping health, building health, having strategies to increase health. The individual becomes an active and participating subject, having the power within themselves, and the ability, to make good choices to avoid falling into the river in the first place. For Antonovsky, we are born in the River of Life (Eriksson and Lindstrom 2008). Some are at the safe end of the river with good resources and opportunities for a good life, but some are at the waterfall end where there are many more risks. We need to develop the ability to identify resources to improve our options for health and life: to learn to swim. Using the life course perspective, we go through transitions in life, and need to develop the ability to manage stress in new situations (Eriksson and Lindstrom 2008), swimming and enjoying the water, not being drowned in distress. Superficially, the use of technology as discussed in chapter 2 can help us develop skills and abilities for health. However, we can only do this in a health-supporting and health-enabling environment with favourable conditions, as described by Green et al. (2015). The challenges lie in how digital technology can be used to foster this supporting and enabling environment.

Reflection 3.1

If you have experience of health promotion practice, which model of health is your practice based on? Can you apply the Salutogenic approach to your practice? How can digital technology help you in your practice?

Implication for practice 3.1

Who are the stakeholders you would collaborate with as a health promotion professsional if you needed to provide your service online? How can you take into account people's economic, social and environmental contexts?

Choice, power, control, participation and empowerment

Empowerment is the process of enabling people to gain some control or power over their lives. We often use the term casually without examining and reflecting whether our actions are really empowering. The overuse and misuse of the term can be seen as cynical, with diminished meaning (Laverack 2013). Power cannot be given. It can only be gained by people who seek it. It involves social relationships.

Laverack (2009) looked at four different types of power:

- Power-from-within is the inner sense of self, an individual gaining control of their own life.
- Power-with is where relationships are equal.
- Powerlessness.
- Power-over – as health professionals, we have power-over our clients that sometimes we may not realize. Raven and Litman-Adizes (1986) identified six forms of power-over that practitioners can have over their clients – *coercive* power, such as legal actions with negative consequences; *reward* power, with positive consequences when a reward is given; *legitimate* power, where an authoritative position may exert influence on others; *expert* power, of being an expert in the field; *reference* power, where the person's characteristics may have influence on others; and *information* power, where the information one holds may give one power over others.

Health promotion is an anti-oppressive activity, working towards social reform and redressing imbalances of power. It is about addressing the cause of powerlessness and disempowerment. People are their own assets, and the role of the external agent is to catalyse and facilitate the community in acquiring power. In many health promotion activities, we often take choice and control as given. You have the choice to stop smoking, the choice to do more exercise, the choice to eat healthy food. But some powerless individuals may have limited choices. There is no doubt that healthy eating and regular exercise are good for health. However, choices are conditioned and constrained by people's living environment. Empowerment is about facilitating voluntary decision making and achieving free choices. We can only make genuine free choices when physical, socioeconomic and cultural circumstances are favourable (Green et al. 2015). Many may not have the knowledge, be too busy working or looking after family, or have inadequate income to make free choices. People need to feel that they have the will, power and capacity within themselves to respond to the environment around them. Freedom of choice, the empowerment of the individual to take control of their health and make informed decisions can sometimes be framed in the context of being a responsible health-conscious citizen in a neo-liberal world where inequality becomes an inevitable outcome – a product of the past and a predictor of the future.

Empowerment can be at individual, organization and community levels. It can also be seen as ranging from individual at one end of the spectrum to collective at the other end. At one end of the spectrum, *individual empowerment* is concerned with self-determination, self-efficacy, self-esteem, self-control – the individual is assumed to have power within themselves to take control over the determinants of their lives. Digital health promotion tends to focus on individual empowerment and relates to the way people think of themselves, including the knowledge, capacities, skills and mastery they actually possess (Staples 1990). At the other end of the spectrum, *collective empowerment* is the process by which individuals join together to break their solitude and silence, help one another, learn together and develop skills for collective action (Boehm and Staples 2004). It is concerned with belonging, being involved and participating, social cohesion, creating a sense of community, increasing the ability to work together, solving problems and making group decision for social change (Mann 2006).

Empowerment at an *organization level* is then about the setting that provides individuals with opportunities to exert control for organizational effectiveness in service delivery and the policy process. At *community levels*, it is how organization(s) and individuals interact to enhance community living and ensure that the community addresses local needs and concerns. Individuals exist within a social system. An empowered community with empowered participating individuals has an active commitment to achieve community goals. Community empowerment is about taking collective action to improve the quality of community life and the connections among organizations, not just about the aggregation of empowered individuals (Zimmerman 2012). Community empowerment is a process of re-negotiating power. It is more than involvement and participation. It implies ownership and action that aims at social and political change (WHO 2009).

As seen in Green et al. (2015), participation and the empowerment gradient are where low degrees of empowerment relate to coercion, with no participation or involvement. High degrees of empowerment link to high levels of participation where members are in control and participating in all decision making. These are fundamental concepts in addressing health promotion in a digital as well as real-world environment. The wide use of Web 2.0 technology has increased the access of information, and opportunities for participation in and contribution to health matters. Superficially, many digital health interventions only focus on individual and lifestyle approaches to promote health, as seen in chapter 2. However, Norman (2012) argues that social media can reduce inequities created by organizations and social position, because everyone functions equally and has an equal voice on the internet, and has opportunities to act on issues on the same platform. This can align with the action areas of the Ottawa Charter. The interactivity and interconnectivity of social media, social networking sites (as well as methods such as tweeting, blogging, etc.) provide a platform for the virtual community to build community empowerment and to enhance mediating, advocating and enabling functions for health promotion.

This takes us to the rhetoric and realities of health. Patient empowerment has been a prominent feature in UK government health policy since the 1980s, as seen in the last ten years' health reform policy documents. By providing information through, for example, the NHS Choices website, and the NHS apps library, patients are empowered to have increased control of their own health. Patients are therefore seeking their own solutions to their own illness. It is important, however, to give words their true meaning. Often the 'right' to choose, the 'right' to give feedback, become 'responsibilities'. Patients being empowered to 'choose' becomes a burden, an obligation; it actually becomes their responsibility to choose (Veitch 2010). Veitch sees patient empowerment as a political technique of governing, to manage the increased costs of healthcare, entrenching the role of the market in healthcare. Through patient empowerment, individuals increase their *self*-responsibility for healthcare, recasting dependency on medical professionals within a marketized model. Competition (the driver of neoliberal markets) is embedded in the healthcare system. Empowerment, increased choice, provision of sound information, increasing control over people's own health and healthcare are simply vehicles for government objectives to promote and establish competitive markets (Veitch 2010).

Words such as 'empowerment' are often misused by professionals, people with power. Pure information provision is not the same as 'critical health education' as described by Green et al. (2015). For example, we often think that by being provided with information, people will have knowledge and be able to make choices: *'information giving'* = *'empowerment'*. 'Independence' means people having to do everything for themselves. But independence is about people having choice and control over all decisions which shape their lives. Laverack (2013) sees the redistribution of power, transforming unequal power relationships within and between societies, as the key to addressing health inequality. Using a Power Analysis framework (Gaventa, 2006; Hunjan and Keophilavong 2010), we can address power at different levels – local, national or international. Power can be seen in different forms: 'visible', where power is explicit; 'invisible', where oppression holds the community back. Power can also be 'hidden' and behind the scenes. There are also different spaces where power can be exercised: 'closed space', where communities are excluded; 'invited space', where communities are invited, be it genuine or manipulated; and there are also 'claimed spaces', which the communities themselves use and own. Empowerment is about enabling participatory person-centred decision making. The Power Analysis framework is a useful framework for practitioners in thinking through their actions (Cross et al. 2017). It is also useful for health promotion practitioners when designing digital health promotion interventions.

Power is multi-dimensional. When there is power, there is counter-power. In a networked society, social power is exercised by and through networks. Castells (2011) discussed four different types of power in a network society:

1 Networking power – the power of those within the network over those outside the network, as seen in network gatekeeping

theory: people who do not add value to the network may be excluded.

2 Network power – the power of the standards, protocols of communication, over the components of the network.

3 Networked power – the power of social actors over other social actors in the network.

4 Network-making power – the power to program specific networks according to the interest and value of the programmers, and the power to switch to a different network.

Empowerment approaches require a lot of reflection on and examination of our own actions, avoiding messages and actions designed to be persuasive, paternalistic, manipulative or coercive – often without us realizing. In using technology to aid health promotion in a networked society, this requires practitioners to examine the power relationships, the environments and the context of their clients. Is the evidence we present to our clients selective? Are they in a position to make a reasonable decision without us influencing them? Have they got the ability, capacity, power within themselves to make that decision? Have they got the information and resources to enable them to make that decision? Are we developing our clients as self-directed thinkers (Mezirow 1997)? For empowerment approaches, the health promoter is a facilitator, a collaborator, a resource for the community, not an expert (Zimmerman 2012). For the health promoter, healthy choices might mean a choice for healthy living. However, for many people, choices might mean that they have to choose whatever is available and suitable for them under their circumstances, because of the social and environmental barriers they face (Cross et al. 2017).

Reflection 3.2

Think of your relationship with your clients – is your approach empowering? If yes, what makes your approach empowering? How do you know your approach is empowering? If not, why not, and how can you change your approach to be more empowering and enabling?

Implication for practice 3.2

If you were asked to design an online health promotion intervention, what would you need to include to ensure that it was empowering? What would your relationship with your clients be like?

Setting approaches to health promotion

Setting approaches in health promotion have been discussed since the 1980s, from the first, third and fourth health promotion conferences. According to the Ottawa Charter statement, 'Health is created and lived by people within settings of their everyday life where they learn, work, play and love' (WHO 1986: 3). It reflects an ecology model of health promotion where health is influenced by a combination of environmental, organizational and personal factors. Ecological whole-system thinking is important in organization development, with inter-relationships and interdependence within and between elements. However, despite many high-profile debates, evidence of its success is limited (Dooris 2005). The challenge is that most research is disease- and risk factor-focused. Some confusion also remains over 'health promotion in a setting', where health promotion interventions were implemented in a setting such as a school or workplace, and the 'setting approach' to health promotion, where health promotion is an *integral part* of the organization and structure of the social system (Baric 1994). There is also confusion on the meaning of a setting (Dooris 2005; Newman et al. 2015). Setting approaches to health promotion mean that the environment and its culture are health promoting – the philosophy of health and policies are embedded in the organization of the setting.

Policies and institutional practices can shape people's opportunities to lead healthy lives. The internet can be used as a 'setting' in cyberspace for health promotion. As described by Loss et al. (2014), given that so much occupational and leisure time is now spent online, online social networks where people can communicate and share information are gaining importance as 'settings' for intervening in health behaviours. Social networking sites as environments for social interaction can be seen as attractive new settings for health promoters. It is a virtual community for many, particularly for young people. However, Loss et al. (2014) are cautious, because of the lack of evaluation and evidence to show how the criteria of setting approaches can be applied within an internet site.

Setting approaches to health promotion can help to improve health and address health inequities (CSDH 2008; Marmot 2010).

Fair Foundations: The VicHealth Framework for Health Equity is a conceptual and planning framework developed by Australia's Victoria Health Foundation (VicHealth 2013). In this framework, social determinants of health inequity are presented as three layers of influences – the socioeconomic, political and cultural contexts; daily living conditions; and individual health-related factors. These determinants and their unequal distribution according to social position result in differences in health status between different population groups, which is avoidable and unfair. In a rapid review, Newman et al. (2015) used this framework to find out how setting approaches can address social determinants of health inequities. Although setting approaches tend to focus on individual health-related factors, there are some initiatives that can address the socioeconomic, political and cultural influences on health – e.g. addressing the structural barriers; ensuring genuine multi-agency participation. There is considerable room for health promoters who use setting approaches to move beyond or integrate individual behaviour approaches in their work.

At present, most online health promotion messages are for individualized behaviour changes, and only a few are on socioeconomic, political and cultural contexts. Many groups are also relatively excluded, e.g. some young disabled people and disadvantaged groups, even with websites intended for universal use. The digital divide will be discussed in chapter 6. In fact, most socio-political factors are outside the control of the healthy settings. In general, there are many opportunities to integrate the individual behaviour approach with approaches at structural and organizational levels. However, structural interventions require more planning, commitment and cross-sectoral collaboration. Upstream interventions to address health inequity logically come first; non-health sectors should be involved. More evidence is also needed for practice. Ten years after Dooris's study on the setting approach to health promotion in 2005, Newman et al. (2015) agree that Dooris's view on the need for funding evaluation still applies.

Implication for practice 3.3
There are many digital health promotion interventions on the web; however, how would you use the 'setting approach' for health promotion via digital technologies in practice? What do you need to consider?

Ethics in digital health promotion

Ethics is a discipline about moral reasoning and moral principles. Health promotion is social and political, and there are different views on what is right and what is wrong. The complexity depends on how health promotion and health are defined (Carter et al. 2012). The normative ideal of health promotion is about equity, equality and social justice. The practice of health promotion as a multi-disciplinary, multi-professional and multi-strategy endeavour covers a wide range of professionals (McPhail-Bell et al. 2015). So it is difficult to determine to whom health promotion ethics apply, and whether we should involve all activities that promote health in ethical consideration. According to Carter et al. (2012), ethics debates in health promotion are more concerned with health promotion practice than with the health promotion normative ideal. Carter et al. (2012) discuss four areas in ethics related to health promotion practice – how health promotion might impinge on the autonomy of the citizen; health promotion as a source of collective benefits; the potential for health promotion practice to cause victim blaming and stigmatizing; and how the benefits of health promotion are distributed fairly in the good society. All these are important issues applicable to digital health interventions.

In public health work, there is often a contradiction between the good of the individual as against the good of the community/society. The contradiction between the empowerment approach, involving personal autonomy, and the paternalistic approach involving persuasion and coercion at the other extreme, can be quite real in health promotion. Indeed, health promotion interventions are often based on balancing the benefits for the collective good as against the respect for individual liberty. Paternalistic coercion cannot always be framed as morally bad. But there is the crucial, but usually unstated, question about who balances the benefits. Who has the final power to, for example, initiate a smoking ban in public places? In a study on health promotion ethics in Australia among the Indigenous community, McPhail-Bell et al. (2015) asserted that health promoters need to recognize their own power at the practitioner and institutional levels over the community that they work with. It's also important for them to recognize the agency of the people, rather than imposing and enforcing their own values on the people they work with. McPhail-Bell et al. argue that health promotion needs explicit discussion of power and its ethical basis. Power sharing with the people whom health promoters work with can contradict the lifestyle-approach agenda. An Individualistic approach may stigmatize those who fail in their 'duty as citizens' to be healthy, with the risk of reinforcing health inequality.

Using obesity as an example, the individualistic paternalistic weight-related public health initiatives online or offline, focusing on physical health outcomes, can cause harm to an individual and raise ethical concerns such as limitations to personal freedoms, coercion, increased moral judgement about food choices and victim blaming, and thus lead to stigmatizing and an increase in health inequities. This type of neoliberal approach in tackling obesity, where the focus is on individual behaviour rather than on structural changes, can lead to people being stigmatized and seen as an economic burden to society (Pause 2017). Within a neoliberal society, fat people are constructed as failed citizens who lack discipline and control. Embracing this type of 'healthism' reinforces fatness as a result of poor choices. The debate on over-weight is not always straightforward. We live in an obesogenic environment where high-calorie food is everywhere, and high-quality food is expensive for many low-income families. There are also other suggested theories on the causes of overweight, such as hormonal effects or biological factors. However, public health campaigns and many digital health promotion activities tend to pay little attention to these social, economic, environmental and structural factors or to consider human rights issues. Individual and lifestyle approaches to health interventions such as those dis-cussed in chapter 2 on digital health promotion can be problem-atic. We should focus not just on individuals' right to health, but also on the right for individuals to be free from being stigmatized for being overweight (Pause 2017). Stigmatizing campaigns are ineffective and increase health disparities. Pause (2017) argues that fat-stigmatizing contributes to the social determinants of health.

A review study by O'Hara et al. (2015) on the ethical issues of Australian weight-related public health initiatives between 2003 and 2013, using the Health Promotion Value and Principles Continuum (Gregg and O'Hara 2007), with ideal critical health promotion practice on one end and common traditional practice on the other, found a wide range of discourses in the reviewed documents on active participation. Documents examined include radio, television, outdoor and online advertisements, and websites. Weight-related interventions are also strongly featured in many digital health promotion programmes. Most participation in the study was low level rather than engaging or involving. The language used in these documents was also strongly professional and controlling, such as 'target group' and 'intervention'. This implicitly takes the powerful 'professional' paradigm as 'correct' and 'scientific'. Even if unintended, this reveals poor understanding of active participation, and can be disabling and disempowering. Overall, there is evidence of discourse supporting moderate active participation in the change process. As regards autonomy, there is a strong discourse of choice. However, it seems that the only choices approvable are healthy choices in an enabling environment. You don't have rights to make bad choices. So, it is an illusion of personal autonomy. The language is paternalistic and the strategy is coercive, involving 'nudging' people to make the 'right' choice. The benefits of these initiatives were overall biomedical. The potential of non-maleficence was rarely raised, and discussion about ineffectiveness was absent. The image the documentaries often portray is about shameful and self-blaming feelings of bad behaviour and being fat. The message is that weight is easily controlled by choosing a healthy lifestyle (calorie in versus calorie out). Evidence presented is thin and selective; discourse on theoretical bases is missing. Evidence on the effectiveness of public health strategies is also limited, and there is a strong need for evidence-based practice. Weight-related public health initiatives reviewed in this study reflected the dominance of the principles and values of traditional, medicalized health promotion, inconsistent with the ethical principles and values of critical health promotion.

O'Hara and Taylor (2018) have reviewed studies on weight-centred health paradigm (WCHP) and call for a paradigm shift from weight-centred to health- and wellbeing-centred. They suggested a Health at Every Size (HAES) model, a weight-inclusive rather than weight-normative model that offers a health-promoting and humane approach to weight concerns. It takes a social justice approach and supports policies, processes and environments that enhance holistic health and well-being, irrespective of shape and size. It urges a focus on social, economic, political and physical environments as underlying determinants of health and wellbeing. Evidence shows this to be more successful than a weight-centric approach (O'Hara and Taylor 2018). As seen from the discussion in the previous sections, WCHP is medical, top-down with a very narrow interpretation of health, and does not really address what public health practitioners set out to address, e.g. tackling the social determinants of health, reducing health inequality or maintaining social justice. It does not mediate or advocate for health as stated in the Ottawa Charter.

Individualistic, lifestyle and behavioural approaches can be seen as blaming people for their poor health. Health promotion strategies that target 'at risk' groups may become stigmatizing. This is not to say that individualized, lifestyle and behavioural approaches are without merit. There is a need for an overall strategy in tackling public health issues and health inequalities. We need to see the full picture and take all factors into account, collaborating with all stakeholders. As seen in Beattie's health promotion model (1991), there are four paradigms in his model, generated from the mode of interventions (authoritative to negotiated) and the focus of interventions (individual to collective). Strategies for health promotion should include health persuasion, legislative action, personal counselling and community development.

Governments need to take a lead and the development of internet technology can be part of this strategy discussion. The public health 'war on obesity' policies and programme have so far had little impact on obesity prevalence (Salas 2015). Ineffectiveness was attributed to a heavy focus on individualized health promotion and behaviour change and health education strategies, ignoring the social–environmental factors, focusing on weight rather than health and failing to take into account the complexity of obesity. Critics argue weight-focused strategies can lead to excessive preoccupation with weight rather than health, which can lead to stigma and weight-related bullying, body dissatisfaction, extreme dieting, depression, low self-esteem, etc., increasing the level of non-maleficence – ethically problematic. In the same way, with digital technology – e.g. wearable devices – Fitbit numbers focusing interventions on physical activity and weight can be detrimental to health in general. Health promoters should avoid over-simplistic messages that focus solely on individual responsibilities.

Health outcomes are important, and strategies should include both individual and system-level determinants of health (Salas 2015; Pause 2017).

Thompson and Kumar (2011) agreed that most health promotion campaigns focused on individual responsibility in a neoliberal context. Behaviour modification campaigns, as seen in many digital health messages, can be seen through the work of the 'governmentality' theorists, where subjects are 'governed at a distance' by being incited to govern themselves (Foucault 1979; Dean 1999). Those who fail to exercise appropriate levels of restraint are subjected to subtle (or unsubtle) forms of self- and/ or social censure. For example, making the right choice can make you a 'good citizen'. Paternalistic health messages can produce resistance. Thompson and Kumar (2011) argue that this process of governance at a distance could be seen as highly contingent and unstable, depending on what we think of as citizenship. Rights and responsibilities were once the marks of citizenship, social responsibility and solidarity with others. However, since the late twentieth century, 'citizenship' reflects the dominance of neoliberal thinking. Empowerment of the individual is good. Citizenship is a contract for individual autonomy with less government intervention, relying on 'governance at a distance' as described by Foucault (Miller and Rose 1993). Participants in Thompson and Kumar's study also indicated that they would like to make their own decisions as whether they want to follow health messages or not, rather than being told what is good for them by the government, – a paternalistic infringement on personal autonomy. Messages lost their effectiveness when people felt that they were being told what to do. Denial is another characteristic response. People don't believe that health messages apply to them. Interestingly, there is also a disapproval of people who don't follow the health advice, which in turn produces stigma in society. There is also the potential for stigmatized individuals further to resist constant health messages, causing a continuing cycle of persecution and resistance (Thompson and Kumar 2011). Thompson and Kumar argue that this stigma associated with non-compliance could further reinforce social inequalities.

Persuasion and coercion strategies can also be paternalistic. Using education approaches which 'encourage/persuade' people to make 'good' decisions can be presented as evidence-based practice and mistaken as empowerment – persuading people to make healthy lifestyle choices; persuading people to consent to screening, vaccination. Public health interventions can range from coercion at one end of the continuum to persuasion and health empowerment at the other end – an ethical-dilemma continuum in health promotion (Hubley and Copeman 2008). At times, it is difficult to recognize when encouragement becomes persuasion and coercion – e.g. financial coercion where health insurance is lower if consumers use wearable health trackers, or employers encouraging their employees to wear health-tracking devices as part of their workplace health initiative (Lupton 2015c).

The Ottawa Charter (1986) can be seen as the cornerstone in health promotion ethics (Sindall 2002; Mittelmark 2007). Authors such as Seedhouse, Sindall, Cribb and Duncan have long discussed health promotion ethics. Health promotion directed at the social determinants of health should focus on populations, not stigmatize individuals or groups. In public health work, the conflict is between the need to prevent disease and safeguard the public's health as against respecting individual freedom of choice, including the freedom to adopt an 'unhealthy' lifestyle. Health promotion as a values-based practice concerned with issues such as empowerment and participation is inevitably bound up with ethical and moral issues. Empowerment means empowering people to make their own 'informed' choices, which may not be the same choices that the health promoters want. Seedhouse (2001) commented that, although there are isolated islands of debate, the quality of discussion around ethical matters in mainstream health promotion is poor.

In a westernized neoliberal context, a libertarian approach privileges the rights of the individual over those of the collective. The assumption is that, once people are informed, they will make good decisions autonomously! Digital technology has emphasized the individual's responsibility for their own health (Lupton 2015c). The principles in traditional biomedical ethics (Beauchamp and Childress 1994) are about autonomy, beneficence, non-maleficence and justice. Traditional biomedical ethics address conflicts at individual levels. Debates such as individual rights versus collective interests can be challenging. The common good may infringe individual liberties and autonomy – for example, infringing on smokers' right and autonomy to smoke, so as to respect non-smokers' rights in smoke-free public spaces. Maintaining a population's health is a complex equation between individuals, organizations and the state, and all have a role to play. Public health work should be contextually and culturally sensitive. It is important for health promotion practitioners to develop the knowledge and skills in ethical reflection on their practice (Cribb and Duncan 2002; Masse and Williams-Jones 2012). In the *Ontario Health Promotion E-Bulletin*, Telford (1998) presented thirteen ethical dilemmas in health promotion practice as adapted from Guttman (1995, 1997). They can also be applied to digital health promotion interventions:

Strategy dilemmas
  1 Persuasion – persuasion in a paternalistic manner can sometimes be seen as empowerment.
  2 Coercion – is it justified to intervene in order to protect others, for example by the use of legislation?
  3 Targeting – targeting certain groups may cause stigmatizing.
  4 Harm reduction – is this a good way forward – e.g. providing needles to drug addicts?

Inadvertent Harm dilemmas
  5 Labelling – which may stigmatize people.
  6 Depriving – e.g., depriving people of the pleasure of smoking
  7 Culpability – who is responsible, the person or the environment? Should some behaviour be permitted, even if others may disapprove?

Power and Control dilemmas
  8 Privileging – does the programme privilege certain stakeholders or ideologies?
  9 Exploitation – does the programme exploit community/voluntary organizations who might support values of participation and empowerment?
 10 Control – does the utilization of programmes and services serve to control their members (e.g., workplace initiatives)?

Social Values dilemmas
 11 Distraction – by emphasizing the importance of certain health-related issues in personal, organizational and societal agendas,

to what extent would this distract people from wider important social issues?

12 Promises – do health campaigners make promises that might not benefit certain individuals / society as a whole?

13 The Health as a Value dilemma – by making health an important social value, would health campaigners promote a certain moralism that might not be compatible with other values?

According to John Stuart Mill's harm principle (Nuffield Council on Bioethics 2007), a person has the autonomy to make decisions regarding their own individual health when the choices they make only affect themselves. For example, arguably, obesity is about an individual's health. However, costs to manage chronic ill health arising from obesity affect everyone. Hence, if the choices made affect more people than the individual, intervention may be necessary for the greater good – for example, in smoking bans. Thus, it is seen as justified that the state has the responsibility for those who are not in a position to make choices. The Stewardship model, a liberal framework proposed by the Nuffield Council on Bioethics (2007: xvi–xvii), provides guidance for decision making on public health intervention, which again can be applied to digital health promotion. According to the Stewardship model, the concerning goals of public health programmes should be to:

- aim to reduce the risks of ill health that people might impose on each other;
- aim to reduce causes of ill health by regulations that ensure environmental conditions that sustain good health, for example by providing clean air and water, safe food and appropriate housing;
- pay special attention to the health of children and other vulnerable people;
- promote health not only by providing information and advice, but also by programmes to help people overcome addictions and other unhealthy behaviours;
- aim to ensure that it is easy for people to lead a healthy life, for example by providing convenient and safe opportunities for exercise;
- ensure that people have appropriate access to medical services; and
- aim to reduce health inequalities.

The constraints of the programmes should:

- not attempt to coerce adults to lead healthy lives;
- minimize interventions that are introduced without the individual consent of those affected, or without procedural justice arrangements (such as democratic decision-making procedures) which provide adequate mandate;
- seek to minimize interventions that are perceived as unduly intrusive and in conflict with important personal values.

The intervention ladder proposed by the Nuffield Council on Bioethics (2007) provides a way of thinking about acceptability. It shows measures from eliminating choice at the top of the ladder, to restricted choice, to guided choice through disincentives, guided choices through incentives, guided choices through changing the default policy, and enabled choice, to providing information, to doing nothing at the bottom of the ladder. It presents a range of options available to policy makers, from individual freedom and responsibility to state intervention. The benefits to individuals and society weigh against the erosion of individual freedom. At times, public health measures can be seen as infringements of liberties, particularly when they become more coercive. There is also the wider ethical concern with the use of digital technology – privacy, confidentiality and data security issues in the Big Data environment. This will be discussed in chapter 5.

Reflection 3.3

Think of an intervention that was delivered online using digital technology, either in your practice or one that you have encountered. What were the ethical dilemmas, if any? At what level was it on the intervention ladder?

Summary conclusion

In this chapter, we challenge many of the assumptions that are made about health, about rights and responsibilities, about 'choice', and about what is ethical in these matters. The chapter has covered health promotion principles and values in relation to the use of digital technology in the public health arena in promoting population health. The complexity of health promotion intertwines with many other professional disciplines. It is almost as complex as the use of digital technology itself. There is great potential for the use of digital technology in public health work via its interactivity and interconnectivity, e.g. in the development of community empowerment, and collaboration with other sectors to overcome social and structural barriers to good health. Contemporary health promotion practice as seen in many digital health messages is based on individualistic lifestyle and behaviour approaches, shaped by the present neoliberal environment. This clearly presents some difficulties for health promoters in meeting the ideals of a social model approach. On the one hand, policy makers do recognize and preach health promotion ideals, but, on the other hand, their actions are aligned with the 'governance at a distance' idea as described by Foucault.

This chapter is about keeping in mind what health promotion is about when going through the rest of this book and when designing health promotion interventions using digital technologies. Digital technology can be a valuable vehicle for health promotion. It is about how we use it, rather than it being individualistic, lifestyle- and behaviour-focused. It is up to the users, the policy makers, the web developers, and the practitioners who work together to enable digital technology as a useful tool and a vehicle for the purpose of health improvement. As current health promotion practice focuses on the individualistic behaviour and lifestyle approach, it is important to look at the underpinning theories that digital health practices are based on – the behaviour theories in the next chapter.

4

Behaviour Change Approach and Behaviour Theories in Digital Health Promotion

Key points

- To discuss the behavioural approach to health promotion in the digital world and consider its effectiveness.
- To consider the theoretical perspectives on behaviour changes, such as behaviour models and self-efficacy, in relation to digital health promotion.
- To explore health behaviour versus health practice.
- To explore social marketing and behaviour change relating to digital health.

Introduction

In seeking to improve health, an understanding of human behaviour is fundamental. This chapter explores the principles of health promotion outlined in the previous chapter more deeply, focusing on individualistic, behaviour and lifestyle approaches to health promotion in the digital world. The evidence on the effectiveness of behaviour change is unclear and there is a wide acknowledgement of the structural causes of poor health and health inequalities. Digitized health promotion as described by Lupton (2013a) tends to focus on self-care and personal responsibility for healthy choices – an individualistic, victim-blaming approach that focuses on lifestyle changes such as physical activities, smoking cessation and dietary choices (Laverack 2017). Similarly, broadly targeted, information-based approaches to promoting health are not always effective in changing behaviour (Mielewczyk and Willig 2007). As already discussed, digital knowledge needs to catch up with health promotion knowledge in this regard.

Linking to previous chapters, the use of digital technologies and the effectiveness of the behaviour/lifestyle approach to promoting health will be discussed in depth. The underpinning theoretical perspectives on behaviour change, such as behaviour models, self-efficacy, and individual motivation and engagement in relation to the use of digital technology, will also be discussed. The focus of the individual behaviour/lifestyle approach in a neoliberal political environment, for health promotion and social marketing strategies, will be explored. The chapter will also consider the concept of 'health practice', health behaviour in the social context – as discussed by Mielewczyk and Willig (2007) and Cohn (2014) – as well as the sustainability and resources needed to support behaviour change, and how digital technologies can enhance individual and community empowerment, complementing health promotion principles and values, linking to the previous chapter.

The behaviour change approach to health promotion in the connected world

Despite the recognition of the social determinants of health (CSDH 2008), the pathogenic medical model of health still dominates, prioritizing illness prevention to avoid pathogenic behaviour. There is a strong belief that digital technology is the cost-effective way to manage healthcare. As already discussed, health promotion using digital technology currently focuses almost exclusively on individual behaviour, ignoring the social–political context of the individual's life. Through our self-caring, self-monitoring processes, we are encouraged to become the ideal citizen, taking responsibility for our own health. The practices of maintaining fitness and self-quantification, as seen in many digital health apps, emphasize this personal behaviour and self-responsibility. Data can be used to help individuals improve their health via feedback from their bodily measurements, which can be sent through mobile devices such as wearable technology. They can also be sent to health professionals who can survey, analyse and monitor our condition in the management of chronic illnesses. With the advance of the Big Data phenomenon and the increasingly sophisticated algorithms to manipulate health-related data, the idea that people should take control of their own health is reinforced.

This approach ignores the fact that some people have limited choice other than using technology in managing their health, for example in chronic health management. Lupton (2013a) gave an example of some US insurance companies incentivizing their clients to use sensor devices such as pedometers as part of their wellness programme to lose weight. The responsibility for care has shifted from government and health professionals to people becoming the ideal responsible citizen and ideal 'digitally engaged patients', as described by Lupton (2012). This is a new neoliberal contract that has gradually shifted society away from welfare rights (1948 – we want a society where support is ensured for everyone who needs it) to consumer obligations (2010s – those citizens who need this support are failed citizens). Those who do not take up the responsibility to improve themselves are seen as failing to achieve the ideal, and it's their own fault for becoming ill (Lupton 2012, 2015c; Horrocks and Johnson 2014).

Within westernized neoliberal society, health is now seen as the individual's responsibility, based on freedom of choice with minimal government intervention and market fundamentalism. The preoccupation of this health consciousness has become part of our capitalist society in what Crawford describes as 'Healthism' (Crawford 1980). Healthism means people taking responsibility to achieve good health, benefitting not only themselves but also society. The burden of health is placed on the consciousness of the individual citizen, rather than the state (Ayo 2010). This phenomenon is facilitated by the rise of a consumerized society in which health-food shops, gyms, exercise equipment and fashion shops sell us goods and services to assist us in the pursuit of good health. Behaviour change becomes an expected way to promote health – the duty and obligation of a responsible self-governing citizen. The growth of digital technologies, such as health apps and social media, fits well into this form of perspective on health. Despite the effort that health promotion has made in the New Public Health era, self-management and self-responsibility in a neoliberal environment lead to those who fail being implicitly presented as ignorant, morally deficient and lacking self-control and the capacity to take appropriate responsibility for their own health (Lupton 2015c).

Ayo discussed five basic neoliberal rationalities that facilitate present-day health promotion discourses and health consciousness: (1) minimal government intervention; (2) market fundamentalism; (3) risk management; (4) individual responsibility; and (5) inevitable inequality as a consequence of choice. These are central to neoliberal politics and highlight the key conflicts between neoliberal principles and the principles underpinning the Ottawa Charter (Ayo 2010). The focus of health policy is now about enabling the individual to make good choices, to take responsibility for their own health. Unemployment, poor housing, low educational attainment, poor transport links ... governments surrender solutions for these to the market. Instead of tackling the social determinants of health, the government encourages free markets – e.g., in the health industry, the public are presented with expert knowledge and guidance on healthy lifestyles and healthy living. Ayo (2010) sees these five tenets of neoliberal society as a symbol of the 'healthy society'. All the messages about healthy eating, being active, reducing the risks of developing chronic ill health and non-communicable conditions become the central focus of health promotion strategies in which people themselves become both the cause and the solution in the management of chronic ill health (Ayo 2010). It's a neo-Victorian mindset – the poor are the object of moralizing; poverty is caused by a weak character; those who rise out of poverty prove the moral weakness of those who remain.

Neoliberal approaches to health can initially be presented as 'choice and control' and 'empowerment'. Seemingly ethical voices advocating on society's behalf become manipulative in order to nudge people into changing their behaviour in the interests of their health. This reduces health problems to a micro-strategy level – focusing on the individual, rather than the structural barriers, increases the stress on the individual (Lupton 2012). It is also important to see choice and control in context – individuals can and do make choices in the context of their surroundings. People can voluntarily and willingly try to improve their own health in their own best interests (Lupton 2015c). Lupton suggests that criticisms about behavioural and lifestyle approaches to health are not about mHealth technology being inherently oppressive and coercive, limiting the individual's agency and freedom, as explained by the writing of Foucault and Deleuze and Guattari. In her view, power is diffuse, spread across many organizations and stakeholders. In a study by Lovell et al. (2014) on the views of health promoters working in a neoliberal climate in New Zealand, where community development approaches are strong, and where contractual arrangements are increasingly common with tight budgets, health promoters found their position inherently ambiguous and inflected with power relations. Given that they are neither agents of the state nor advocates for the community, they work in collaboration with the community strategically to achieve health promotion goals and mitigate the unwelcome effects of competition in the public health system.

In the age of austerity, individualistic and lifestyle approaches can be a cheaper option for healthcare, as compared with tackling the social determinants of health. Digital technologies allow ways to target certain individuals with tailored messages, and to monitor their body functions. Health and wellbeing become numbers collected from tracking devices, game apps or sensor-embedded objects (Lupton 2015c). Lupton (2013a) calls this present-day digital health revolution in health promotion 'digitized health promotion'. Despite the efforts that health promoters have put into the concepts of health and the importance of the social determinants of health since the 1970s, digital technology has renewed/reinforced a neoliberal concept of health, promoting individual responsibility for it. According to Lupton (2015c), digitized health promotion renders people's health even more individualized, drawing attention away from the social determinants of health to a greater degree than ever before. Policy makers consciously intend the state to self-absolve and shift any burden to its citizens, even though the same policy makers reference the social determinants of health as their context for policy-making documents.

The use of behaviour change approaches in digital health and their effectiveness

Using obesity as an example, childhood obesity and the reduction of physical activity are global causes for concern that lead to many non-communicable diseases such as circulatory diseases, Type 2 diabetes, etc. The exposure of children and young people to food and drink marketing may be underestimated when only traditional broadcasting media are taken into account. Children are less able to differentiate advertising on websites, as compared with that on television (Blades et al. 2013). Food advertisements can be categorized into four areas – broadcasting via television and radio; non-broadcasting via print, cinema, online and social media channels; in-store advertisement, such as product packaging; and advertising under the guise of commercial partnerships and sponsorship – e.g. in sport and cultural events. According to Public Health England (2015), there is strong evidence that the marketing of food containing High Fat, Sugar and/or Salt (HFSS) contributes to children's food choices and consumption practice. A strategic counterbalance to this is that settings where children and adolescents gather (e.g. school, cultural events, sporting events) and screen-based programmes they watch should be free from unhealthy food (WHO 2016).

In the UK, the food industry spent more than £250 million in 2014 on promoting 'unhealthy' food. The spending on junk food advertising is nearly thirty times what government spends on promoting healthy eating (O'Dowd 2017). In the USA, a total of $4.6 billion was spent on all advertising by fast-food restaurants in 2012, and McDonald's spent 2.7 times as much to advertise its products as all fruit, vegetable, bottled water and milk advertisers combined (Yale Rudd Centre 2013). New media – such as the internet, social media and mobile phones – create new avenues for food and beverage companies to communicate with children and young people. In an audit of new media produced by the three top-selling food and beverage brands in Australia, Boelsen-Robinson et al. (2015) found that child-targeted marketing is evident. Engagement techniques of flash animation, games and music were often used for promotional activities aimed at children, and techniques such as viral marketing were aimed at adolescents. Healthy messages tend to appear infrequently, and often focused on physical activities rather than nutrition.

Internet-based behaviour change interventions can be effective. However, there is a big variation in their success, depending on different combinations of design features (Mielewczyk and Willig 2007; Michie et al. 2012; Cohn 2014; Morrison et al. 2014). There is little detail on the content and principles used in the development of these interventions. Evaluation of behaviour change interventions is often rare, inadequate or inadequately shared. In developing effective behavioural change internet-based interventions, psychological theory, evidence of effectiveness, principles of web design and user testing are important. The digital divide is also important in ensuring disadvantaged groups are not excluded (Michie et al. 2012).

The use of behaviour change techniques and behaviour change theory in technology-enabled interventions happens in varying degrees. A comprehensive review by Winter et al. (2016) on cardiovascular disease prevention and treatment in adults found that internet platforms and mobile phone apps are most frequently used. New technologies such as virtual realities, gaming and avatars are used in 'cue reactivity' in tobacco use, increasing mobility in stroke patients, physical activity and weight management, virtual coaching for diet management, social media for social support. The most frequently used behaviour change techniques were self-monitoring, and feedback on performance. Other techniques, such as information provision, goal setting, problem solving and action planning, are also used. Only half of the articles reviewed named a behaviour theory or model. The most frequently used theories were social-cognitive theory, the trans-theoretical model, and the theory of planned behaviour / reasoned action. Innovative design of the programme, combined with theory and evidence, are needed to optimize health promotion interventions (Winter et al. 2016). There is a need to assess effectiveness and cost-effectiveness of mHealth interventions for behaviour change, as compared with other strategies (Thirumurthy and Lester 2012). A better understanding of behaviour change techniques and technology channels is needed.

Behaviour theories such as control theory and social cognitive theory advocate the use of feedback. Providing feedback is important for learning and is central in two-way interactive communication. Understanding theories helps to explain how feedback works in behaviour change interventions. Control theory is about self-regulation for goal-directed behaviour (e.g. walking 10,000 steps per day). Thus, negative evaluation where the recipient's goal has not been met would be likely to increase the effort to perform. Performance would be maintained or decrease with positive evaluation where one has already achieved the goal (Kramer and Kowatsch 2017). However, according to social-cognitive theory, the perception of behaviour and a standard is not enough to regulate behaviour – rather, social cognition, such as self-efficacy beliefs, is central to goal pursuit and self-regulation. A person's self-efficacy influences their goal setting and commitment. When a person has strong self-efficacy, believing s/he has capabilities, s/he will succeed. Thus, positive evaluation will increase self-efficacy, and in turn increase performance. Negative evaluation represents failure, which undermines confidence in one's ability to achieve goals and will in turn decrease performance. A study on using feedback by email to promote physical exercise, by Kramer and Kowatsch (2017), found that there was no difference between the effect of positive and of negative feedback. This, however, could be due to the way feedback was given in their study, in which a feedback email was given only once a month and the authors did not check whether the emails were received. The relevance of the feedback messages may also have been compromised as the recipients could receive feedback from their own exercise-tracking devices. Personalized messages could also have enhanced the relevance of the feedback messages. Feedback characteristics should therefore be carefully considered when providing feedback. Using Web 2.0 technologies, such as wearables and mobile phone apps with built-in sensors, personalized feedback messages can be sent when encouragement is needed.

Tailoring feedback and user support – e.g. via self-assessment, monitoring, planning and goal setting – are commonly used design features, and tailoring seems to be more engaging than generic interventions, in which only information and advice are provided on the internet pages – a two-way interactive communication versus one-way communication. A study on the effect of self-assessment and tailored feedback by Morrison et al. (2014) showed that using self-assessment on health conditions without receiving tailored feedback is less acceptable for participants and has a greater dropout rate. Without feedback, self-assessment offered no benefit. Self-assessment without tailored feedback was also marginally less engaging, and led to fewer positive perceptions than just providing generic information only. Patient engagement is important in healthcare, and real-time communication and feedback are considered essential in supporting behaviour change and empowering patient engagement. Digital technology can offer healthcare professionals more opportunities to engage with people, vis-à-vis traditional face-to-face contact. However, the effectiveness of digital technology on patient engagement and behaviour change was unclear. A systematic review by Sawesi et al. (2016) found that interventions using digital technology had a great impact on patient's health outcomes through patient engagement. However, few studies address the usability of these interventions. The reasons for not using behaviour theories were also unclear.

Innovation in mHealth is also evident in the Global South. For example, two studies in Kenya on the use of text messaging by mobile phone to improve adherence to antiretroviral therapy (ART) for people living with HIV infection have proven to be successful and to prolong viral suppression (Thirumurthy and Lester 2012). One study was based on a weekly two-way text communication, which was successful, and another on a one-way text-message reminder – weekly in one group, and daily in another. There was a higher ART adherence with the group receiving weekly messages than those receiving daily messages. The weekly periodic reminder appeared to be useful as supportive communication for behaviour change. Both studies demonstrated the cost-effectiveness of the interventions: although the use of two-way communication where feedback and interaction are available is slightly more expensive than the one-way communication method where there is no interaction, the cost represents only a fraction of the cost of ART. There is a need for comparison with other more traditional interventions, such as home visits. Other variables also need to be taken into account – e.g. setting-up and implementing costs, specific groups of people, health literacy issues. There are many factors influencing people's adherence to drug regimens; other mHealth strategies such as health apps, social media platforms other than text messaging, as well as sustainability of behaviour changes, also need consideration. In many developing countries, other than in interventions around HIV infection, mHealth can be useful for areas such as maternal and child health; better electronic communication is also useful for health providers.

In a review by Webb et al. (2010) on the importance of theoretical foundations, the use of behaviour change techniques and mode of delivery for efficacy, more extensive use of theory was associated with a bigger impact. There is frequent use of social-cognitive theory, the transtheoretical model, the theory of reasoned action, and theory of planned behaviour. However, the use of theory of planned behaviour in intervention design showed a more substantial effect as compared with other theories. Similarly, behaviour change techniques used were also linked to impacts – e.g. stress management and general communication skills training were associated with greater changes, via problem solving, promoting self-efficacy or stressor reduction. They also found that the use of text messaging and access to an advisor providing personal contact also improved effectiveness. There is considerable variability in the effectiveness of internet-based interventions. A theoretical basis for interventions is recognized as important by many. However, it is unclear whether and how theory can influence intervention effectiveness, particularly with digital health. Practitioners also need to understand the use of different theories and different models, as all theories and models have their own strengths and weaknesses.

Reflection 4.1

If you have experience as a health promotion professional, is your health promotion practice behaviour-focused? Is there any area of your work that focuses on structural factors that influence health? Can you give three examples?

Implication for practice 4.1

Thinking of health promotion practice in relation to behaviour change – how could digital technology help you in practice?

Theoretical perspectives of the behaviour change approach – behaviour models

Justifications for study of health behaviour interventions in health promotion are based on two assumptions – that deaths in industrialized countries are strongly related to particular behaviour patterns, and that these patterns are modifiable; therefore changing one's behaviour should be an effective way to promote health (Conner and Norman 2015; Laverack 2017). Social cognitive models are commonly used to explain health behaviour. Social cognition is concerned with how individuals make sense of social situations. It is believed that social cognition determinants are important in health behaviour and are open to change. (Conner and Norman 2015). Self-regulation, involving people enacting their self-conceptions, enables behaviour change or environment change to achieve people's personal goals. It consists of motivation and volition. Many social cognition behaviour models are concerned with motivation, rather than the volition of the self-regulatory process (Conner and Norman 2015).

One type of social cognition model concerns explanation of events. It focuses on response to illness, rather than to health in general. A second type is about prediction of health-related behaviour and outcomes, e.g. the Health Belief Model, protection motivation theory, the theory of reasoned action and the theory of planned behaviour. Human behaviour is assumed to be rational. There is also a different set of models focused on different stages of behaviour change – e.g., the transtheoretical model of change, which can be applied alongside other models. Change occurs in stages. Individuals go through different stages of change to achieve behaviour goals. Each stage is a step towards achieving a change in behaviour. It is useful to look at the features of some of these commonly used models.

Box 4.1 shows just some features of a few such models. If you want to learn more, please refer to health promotion or behaviour theory texts that can provide detailed critiques.

There have been few strong comparative studies to show how different models compare with each other. Most studies reported similar predictive power between the models and underlying constructs. Considering the large amount of overlap between constructs and the models, there is an agreement among prominent theorists that there is a need to develop an integrated approach (Conner and Norman 2015). Bandura (2004) argued that there are many overlaps in psychosocial health behaviour models. For example, in the Health Belief Model (Becker 1984; Janz and Becker

Box 4.1 Some popular behaviour models

Health Belief Model (HBM) (Becker 1984; Janz and Becker 1984)	This was developed for the prediction of people's adoption of preventative health behaviours, and behavioural responses to medical treatment. Decision making depends on individuals believing that a particular course of action will result in the likelihood of a valued outcome. HBM assumes rational decision-making behaviour, weighing up the pros and cons based on people's perceptions of risk, consequences and perceived benefits and disadvantages. Decisions about health behaviour also depend upon the person's knowledge and experience and any external cues for action. The model requires the person's confidence in making the change. It helps to visualize the basis of a particular health behaviour decision.
Theory of planned behaviour (TPB) (Ajzen 1991) and theory of reasoned action (TRA) (Ajzen and Fishbein 1980)	The TPB outlines factors influencing a person's intention to perform a behaviour. It is an extension of the TRA model, in which people's intention to perform a certain health behaviour is based on our judgement of the balance of the person's attitude – the beliefs about the consequences of taking action, judgement of those consequences, and subjective norms (approval and disapproval from others). The TPB was based on the TRA, with the person's perceived behaviour control as an added element. It includes both the person's internal and external environmental control factors (which influence the intention) and their behaviour outcomes. However, the concept of the subjective norm was criticized as too restrictive – the construct was narrowly focused and less consistent in explaining variance in outcomes than other predictor variables. Perceived behaviour control was also seen as an inferior predictor of self-efficacy. The reliance on intentions rather than behaviour as a measure of outcome is also a methodological weakness. The theoretical, methodological and performance-based weaknesses meant that the social cognitive model failed to take into account the complex nature of health behaviour and was viewed as not fit for purpose by authors such as Mielewczyk and Willig (2007).
Protection motivation theory (PMT) (Rogers 1975)	The PMT is a model exploring how fear appeals work and direct activities to protect oneself from danger. It describes the adaptive and maladaptive responses to a threat through one's threat appraisal and coping appraisal mechanisms. Threat appraisal involves the assessment of the severity of threat to health, and vulnerability to that threat. The coping appraisal mechanism assesses personal efficacy – to see whether the person has the ability to take action – and the response efficacy – to see whether the person has the ability to act on the recommendations to reduce the threat. Hence, for health promotion interventions to be effective, solutions to health threats need to be in place to *(cont.)*

Box 4.1 (continued)

Protection motivation theory (PMT) (Rogers 1975)	help people along the way. Threatening people with the consequences of risk factors – e.g., the dangers of smoking, drinking or casual sex – without providing solutions and advice would be counter-productive, as people might just treat the health messages as irrelevant.
Elaboration likelihood model (ELM) (Petty and Cacioppo 1986)	The ELM is about persuasion for attitude change, to explain different ways health messages are processed. It proposes two major routes to persuasion: the central systematic route, where there is a greater cognitive elaboration; and the peripheral route, where message processing is superficial with a low cognitive processing of messages. People use simple rules to evaluate messages – for example: Expertise equals Accuracy, Consensus equals Correctness. People are more likely to engage in central route processing if they see the message as personally relevant. We are all different. Some of us think more deeply. When there is a lack of time or there are distractions or if we don't understand something, we may only process messages superficially. We may also trust messages if the source is believed to be an expert. 'Low relevance' people are strongly affected by perceived expertise and more persuaded by an expert source, and 'high relevance' people are persuaded by the quality of the argument. Hence, health promotion messages should encourage systematic processing, be easily understood, and have a strong evidence base, emphasizing a personal relevance.
Transtheoretical model (TTM) (Prochaska and DiClemente 1984)	The TTM is a stage-of-change model – individuals are at different change stages. This is a popular model among practitioners. It consists of five different stages – pre-contemplation of change, contemplation of change, ready to change, action, and maintenance of the change. A person may be at any stage of change; they may enter or exit at any stage. After a period of maintenance, the individual may relapse. The process is cyclic. From a social cognition perspective, different cognition may be important at different stages, and different interventions may be appropriate at different stages. Interventions are individually tailored. Assessment is made to determine which stage the individual is at. Self-efficacy plays a role in the individual determining where s/he has the confidence to make the change.

1984), perceived severity and susceptibility to disease predict negative physical outcomes, and perceived benefits lead to positive outcome expectations. In the theory of reasoned action (Ajzen and Fishbein 1980) and theory of planned behaviour (Ajzen 1991), attitudes towards behaviour and social norms produce intentions that determine behaviour. Attitudes are measured by perceived outcomes. Norms are measured by perceived social pressure. Intentions are proximal goals. The perceived control overlaps with self-efficacy. These health behaviour models are concerned with predicting health habits, explaining decision making. They don't actually show people how to change their health behaviour, whereas social cognitive theory offers both predictors and principles on how to guide and motivate people to adopt health behaviour (Bandura 2004).

Health behaviour also depends on what people think the outcome of their action would be, including physical outcomes such as pleasurable and aversive effects, and accompanying material losses and benefits; social outcomes, such as social approval and disapproval; and personal outcomes, such as self-evaluation. People regulate behaviour according to self-evaluation, maintaining their personal standards, self-satisfaction and self-worth. Helping people to see the benefits of change can enhance motivation. Personal goals are value based. Long-term goals help people to set the course for personal change. However, it's difficult to see long-term achievement in a busy life. Setting short-term goals is easier to help people deal with their current situation.

The use of theoretical underpinning for behaviour change interventions can improve design and practical applications. It provides a means for identifying appropriate targets for interventions. In the practice field, many interventions are not theoretically based, and it is unclear whether use of theory does improve the effectiveness of interventions. Most models provide an incomplete understanding of behaviour change and oversimplify the behaviour change process. They focus on beliefs, goals and plans and pay little attention to the capability and opportunity needed for behaviour change to occur. They also ignore the social, cultural and environmental context. Research on health behaviour also rarely looks at theories involving automatic processes, such as drive, emotions, habits and impulses (Conner and Norman 2015).

Reflection 4.2

If you have experience as a health promotion professional, do you use behaviour models for your practice? How useful or otherwise is it to use models to help with your practice?

Implication for practice 4.2
Choose two behaviour models mentioned above, and discuss how they can be applied to health promotion practice.

Theoretical perspectives of the behaviour change approach – self-efficacy

The core determinants in Bandura's social cognitive theory include knowledge of the health risk and benefits of different health practices, our perceived self-efficacy in controlling our health habits, outcome expectations of the cost and benefits for different health habits, health goals people set for themselves, their plans and strategies for achieving these goals, perceived facilitators, and the social and structural impediments to achieving goals (Bandura 2004). Knowledge of health risks and benefits is a catalyst for change. Self-influences are needed to overcome obstacles and enable change. And self-efficacy plays a central role in the process of change. This personal efficacy is the foundation of human motivation and actions. Motivation to change is rooted in the core belief that one has the power to change. Social cognitive approaches to health are about promoting effective self-management of our health habits and keeping people healthy (Bandura 2004). This is important as demand for health services, and costs, increase with an ageing population.

Self-efficacy is key to social cognitive theory and many health behaviour models. It can affect people's behaviour directly or, via the person's intention, indirectly. The focus of self-efficacy is on the notion of human agency, a feeling of having the capacity to influence situations. 'Self-efficacy' means people's beliefs about their capabilities to produce designated levels of performance, exercising influence over events that affect their lives – a perception of their ability to perform a behaviour (Bandura 1977). People with high self-efficacy believe in their abilities to achieve higher goals, have stronger commitment, expect better outcomes and can face difficult challenges. They believe in their self-management skills and perseverant efforts. According to Bandura, people with a high sense of self-efficacy and positive outcome expectations can achieve behaviour change with minimal guidance, whereas those with self-doubt need additional support through tough times.

Those believing their health habits are beyond their personal control would need a lot of personal guidance and motivation to build their efficacy progressively.

Behaviour- and lifestyle-change health promotion interventions, such as those used in digital health promotion, rely on people's high self-efficacy for self-management and positive outcome expectations. Self-regulatory skills and motivation are important for change to happen. Various strategies – such as information provision, shock tactics, increasing perception of risk and raising one's self-efficacy – can be used to help the change process. With the advance of interactive digital technology, tailored health messages can be sent to individuals. Social support and guidance that increase self-efficacy can also be provided through online communities. Interactive personalized feedback can help motivate, guide and enable people through the change process. From a societal point of view, population-based campaigns can also be used – e.g., via the use of social media and social networking sites.

Bandura (2004) asserted that individualist approaches and structuralist approaches to health are not mutually exclusive. Health promotion needs both. The health of a nation is a social as well as personal matter. It requires changing the practice of a social system as well as the habits of the individual. This is similar to the concept of social practice, as discussed by Cohn (2014) and Mielewczyk and Willig (2007). Collective efficacy is needed for a social approach to work. Collective efficacy refers to a group's shared belief in its capability to organize and execute actions required to achieve goals. The focus of a social approach is on collective enablement for changing social matters, a process which equips people with the beliefs and means to produce effects through their collective action. It is about changing the political and environmental conditions that affect health, raising awareness of health hazards, educating and influencing policy makers, building community capacity to change health policy and practice, and mobilizing collective citizen action to override vested political and economic interests. Bandura argued that social cognitive theory extends the conception of human agency to collective agency. We can work together, share beliefs in a collective efficacy to accomplish social change – e.g., the enablement of an online community self-help using social networking sites. He called for an ambitious socially orientated agenda of research and practice with the assistance of evolving interactive technologies. This aligns with health promotion ideals and practice.

Health behaviour versus health practice

As chronic ill health and non-communicable disease epidemics continue, health behaviour (as a topic, and as a concept for health studies and health promotion interventions) remains a common discussion. When we discuss health behaviour, the focus is on poor health behaviour, poor lifestyles that lead to poor health – a *negative* concept in terms of promoting good health behaviour in order to prevent ill health: a *medical* concept, a pathological condition that causes ill health. Social cognition models, as discussed above, fail to take into account the affective factors, even though emotional factors play a part in the decision-making process. Although there has been a lot of discussion on social cognition models for explaining and predicting health behaviour, the studies in this area tend to focus on the intervention itself, its theoretical underpinning, or issues with implementation or outcome measurement, and rarely on the concept of health behaviour itself (Mielewczyk and Willig 2007; Cohn 2014).

As seen in many digital health promotion interventions, in focusing on the behavioural cause of ill health, interventions to promote health are about avoiding pathogenic behaviour, and modifying people's health beliefs, attitudes and behaviours, with self-efficacy as an important element in achieving good health behaviour. Health management and maintenance are solely achieved by self-management and self-regulation. Thus, it becomes a victim-blaming approach – personal weakness causes poor health (Lupton 2012; Horrocks and Johnson 2014). Mielewczyk and Willig (2007) and Cohn (2014) argue that social cognition models are no longer fit for purpose. People are not always rational decision makers, and health psychology fails to address the nature of health behaviour, the relevance of social context, and simplistic quantification of health-related activities (Horrocks and Johnson 2014). In discussing individual health behaviour without the context, other health-related activities – such as what people do in different situations – are ignored. The social, affective, material and interrelational elements are not taken into account. Citing a series of articles demonstrating that the concept of health behaviour is far removed from lived experience, Cohn (2014) argued that reconceptualizing what people do in terms of health practices would be useful in capturing people's activities in context, not to replace health behaviour as a concept, but to allow more freedom for understanding human behaviour. Mielewczyk and Willig (2007) also argue that there is a need to focus on wider social practices. However, public health policy in a neoliberal environment tends to focus on individual responsibility and fails to take into account *either* the wider systemic and structural determinants of health *or* the complex relational settings in which behavioural practices take place. It assumes a reflexive, health-conscious individual, willing and able to make appropriate 'choices' (Crawshaw 2013).

We behave differently in different situations. Meaning and context are important. To understand the motivation that drives the adoption of certain health behaviour, we need to know the practices of which these behaviours form a part (Mielewczyk and Willig 2007). For example, using condoms may communicate a lack of trust for some in a stable long-term relationship when other forms of contraception are available. Thus, there is a need to understand the context and the meaning when condoms are used. Similarly, behaviour may be perceived differently in different contexts. For example, drinking at a celebratory event may be different from drinking at home in the evening. It is easier to adopt protective health behaviour within one context, but more difficult in another. Understanding context and meaning may help researchers or practitioners understand the motivations that drive behaviour. Practitioners need to take into account these contexts in designing digital health promotion interventions.

With the variation in contexts and meaning, robust study of health-related behaviour within the framework of social cognitive models is limited (Mielewczyk and Willig 2007). In health-related research, it may be more constructive to focus on wider social practices in which the specific behaviour forms a part – for example, a narrative approach to research might be a better way to understand the complexity of human behaviour. Understanding the meaning and context also helps practitioners develop tailored interventions, rather than a one-size-fits-all approach to health promotion. For example, client-centred or group activities may be more useful to help people in adopting healthy behaviour, or to suggest other activities to replace the unhealthy one in certain contexts. Unsurprisingly, the change of one's behaviour can also involve the change of one's identity – a new self emerges, for example a non-smoker now was previously a smoker. Health promotion practitioners need to be sensitive to the change in their client's sense of self and identity, which may impact on the readiness for change. With the development of Web 2.0 technology in digital health, interactivity is an advantage in enabling more appropriate interventions. For example, when using social media and social networking sites, incorporate discussions, comments and feedback, building an online community where people have similar social backgrounds, to share experience and support for each other.

Reflection 4.3

Thinking of your own work experience – would you say you focus on individuals' health behaviour rather than health practice? Can you cite three examples of your work experience that focus on health practice rather than health behaviour? How do you take into account your clients' social context when designing digital health promotion activities? If you do not yet have experience as a health promotion professional, how would you plan to take into account your clients' social context when designing digital health promotion activities?

Social marketing and the behaviour change approach

Social marketing was originally discussed and given a name in the 1960s by Kotler and Levy (1969), and later in 1971 by Kotler and Zaltman on applying standard marketing principles with the aim of achieving social good – an approach to planned social change. The primary focus is on the consumer. Early social marketing examples include family planning programmes in Sri Lanka, oral rehydration projects in Africa as part of international development efforts, as well as heart health and high blood pressure prevention in the developed world (MacFadyen et al. 1999). Although Kotler and Zaltman 'invented' social marketing, the early meaningful definition was from Andreasen (1995): the application of commercial marketing technologies to the analysis, planning, execution and evaluation of programmes designed to influence the voluntary behaviour of target audiences in order to improve their personal welfare and that of their society. Social marketing is 'an approach used to develop activities aimed at changing or maintaining people's behaviour for the benefit of individuals and society as a whole' (Hopwood and Merritt 2011: 40). It 'seeks to develop and integrate marketing concepts with other approaches to influence behaviours that benefit individuals and communities for the greater social good' (iSMA, ESMA and AASM 2013: 1).

According to the National Social Marketing Centre (n.d.), the social marketing benchmark criteria are:

- behaviour – aims to change people's actual behaviour;
- exchange, whereby the consumers need to pay a price, such as time or discomfort associated with the change of behaviour, in exchange for benefits that the consumers value – for example, good health;
- audience segmentation where people are differentiated into subgroups;
- competition – seek to understand what competes for the audience's time, attention and inclination to behave in a particular way;
- consumer orientation – focuses on the audience's need, their behaviour and social contexts;
- insight – consumer research identifies actionable insights;
- theory – uses behaviour theories to understand behaviour and inform interventions; and
- the marketing mix concept, which consists of the four Ps – Product/services, Promotion, Place/location of service, and Price.

In addition,

- Weinreich (2006) also included four additional Ps – Publics, Partnership, Policy and Purse strings.

In the short term, social marketing is about the use of marketing strategies such as persuasion and impression management to provide services using marketing techniques to connect to buyers. In the long term, it is about creating products that people need, reaching out to customers (Chriss 2015). Despite the wide use of social marketing strategies, Grier and Bryant (2005) argued that health promoters do not completely understand how social marketing works. Many health promoters often perceive social marketing as a promotional or communicational activity, creating the misconception that social marketing uses mass media advertising alone to achieve its goal, neglecting all other elements in the marketing mix concept (Grier and Bryant 2005; Dibb 2014). Some also see it as a 'nudge-based' intervention. Unlike education approaches or legislation, social marketing aims to create an environment more conducive for change – it influences behaviour change by offering choices, and invites voluntary exchange. Social marketing focuses on individual behaviour change. However, Grier and Bryant (2005) assert that the target audience can include policy makers addressing broader social and environmental determinants of health. In reality, it is primarily still behavioural change, downstream-focused, and a victim-blaming neoliberal approach – and rarely sees policy makers as the target audience.

Some argue that social marketing is manipulative. Using terms such as 'target audience', 'customers', it ignores participatory principles of health promotion. Health promotion theory focuses more on creating a supportive environment to enable the adoption of healthy behaviour, not on changing people's behaviour using persuasive manipulation as a primary goal (Grier and Bryant 2005; Gordon et al. 2016). More recently, there have been signs of social marketing broadening its scope to focus more on upstream health promotion, disrupting the environment and involving stakeholders bringing about social changes – for example, legislative and regulatory changes on drinking, smoking and food consumption (Dibb 2014). Upstream social marketing has been generally welcomed, but there are challenges – e.g. those who don't really embrace the need to develop ideas or those who have a rather dated, 'advertising' understanding of the discipline (Dibb 2014).

Social marketing is about enabling social change by tackling 'wicked problems' (Gordon et al. 2016: 1059). It is said to be effective at a population level across a range of public health issues, e.g. smoking and nutrition. Persuasive messages are more effective when health communication messages are tailored to the target audience. However, persuasive manipulation can have unintended consequences, such as stigmatization. To enable social marketing to achieve social changes (compared with, and complementary to, other methods), training and education on the understanding of principles and implementation as well as research methodologies are needed. Discussion about social good depends on an ethical perspective. Ethical dilemmas and decision making, the issues of choice and control and the issues of empowerment also apply to social marketing. Ethically, marketing of social products is different from commercial marketing – it involves our beliefs and moral judgements as well as unequal power differentials between marketers and consumers (Grier and Bryant 2005). Participatory approaches, with the collaboration of all stakeholders, including the people, are important in addressing the power differentials throughout the whole process (Andreasen 2003; Grier and Bryant 2005).

In order to promote health and social change effectively upstream, there is a need to go beyond individual behaviour change. As social marketing matures, there remain debates on similarities and differences between social and commercial marketing. Appropriate theoretical frameworks beyond individual psychology and economic theory need to include social, cultural and critical theory to understand and ensure the continuous development of social marketing (Grier and Bryant 2005; Dibb 2014; Gordon et al. 2016). Needs assessment and programme evaluation with appropriate methodologies are important to inform programme planning (Grier and Bryant 2005). It is also important that social marketers face the challenges, engaging debate with reflexivity, and work with other disciplines and stakeholders, including people and communities, collaboratively (Dibb 2014; Gordon et al. 2016). As discussed above regarding the effectiveness of the behaviour approach to health promotion, a combination of different approaches and strategies to behaviour change in health promotion is advisable (Dibb 2014). Critical and inclusive debate is needed, including a diversity of voices from different ethnic, sociocultural and gender perspectives (Gordon et al. 2016).

Social marketing and digital health

As interconnectivity increases, mobile marketing becomes a new opportunity for health promotion (Thackeray et al. 2008, 2012; Lefebvre 2009; Coiera 2013; Dibb 2014). Digital technologies could facilitate engagement of, and foster partnerships with, the public (Coiera 2013). Promotion through the different functions of mobile technologies is also very useful because of the interconnectivity, and the access to two-way communication with service providers. Digital interventions, as discussed in chapter 2, can motivate and offer support and feedback, and reach further into people's everyday lives (Chou et al. 2013). Connected consumers can be segmented into different groups by the way they use their mobile devices, rather than the traditional demographic attributes. Through the use of the internet, behaviour change products and services are readily available via social media and social networking sites. For people to engage in new behaviour, the price of the intervention is financial, psychological and social, such as cost, privacy and confidentiality. Digital devices have unexplored possibilities as long as there is access to mobile networks. Mobile devices become marketing tools that address all elements of the marketing mix and provide opportunities for health promoters and social marketers (Lefebvre 2009; Dibb 2014). The interconnectivity and interactiveness of Web 2.0 technology can help achieve viral marketing at high speed (Thackeray et al. 2008). Data capture also helps in gathering personal and behavioural information for market trends and market research, as well as for needs assessment. It helps in measuring and monitoring of personal activity, as well as intervention development. Data can also be gathered for a particular region or community, or people with specific conditions (Dibb 2014).

Social marketing was used by the UK government in the form of the Change4Life campaign to tackle obesity in 2011. The then Secretary of State for Health, Andrew Lansley, accepted the impact of environmental and social factors on health and wellbeing, and health inequalities, and at the same time posited individual behaviour as the key for improving health. Lansley described the Change4Life social marketing campaign as a 'new social movement' (Crawshaw 2013: 6), drawing the community and voluntary sectors together, as well as working with commercial sectors in promoting healthy choices and behaviours. In contrast to the Marmot review recommendations (2010), with social marketing and the increased use of digital technologies, people can easily be 'nudged' to make the right choice ('Nudge' as a concept and a policy tool will be discussed in chapter 6, 'Digital Technology and Health Inequality').

Social marketing works on the assumption that people can and should take responsibility for their own health. In a study on the understanding of social marketing among senior public health practitioners, Crawshaw (2013) found that there is a good understanding of social marketing among this group, who are comfortable with the approach. There is a clear recognition of the tension between the individual behaviour-change approach and the structural determinants of health; practitioners also accepted social marketing as a credible approach to behaviour change, although they also recognized the difficulties in changing behaviour as compared with selling goods in a commercial market. Similarly, with choices and responsibility, people have the responsibility, and should be able to make informed choices, for their own health. There is also an understanding of the contextual constraints and the complexity of making choices. Crawshaw's study shows the acceptance of the individualistic approach of neoliberalism in the world of public health among professionals, even though they recognize the social and environmental contexts that influence individuals' behaviour choices (Crawshaw 2013).

Starting with the Black Report in 1980 (DHSS 1980), and continuing to the Marmot Review (Marmot 2010), as well as WHO documents on social determinants of health (CSDH 2008), there is a recognition of the widening gap of health and social inequalities. However, the individualist behaviour-change approach remains – partly because it can be appropriate for promoting health, partly because neoliberalism is an unavoidable reality. The popular strategic use of social marketing demonstrates the entrenchment of neoliberalism in society. With the short interval between governmental elections, behaviour change is attractive to policy makers as it promises cost-effective short-term results (Laverack 2017). It also aligns with the reality that governments are unlikely to implement bolder structural changes to improve health, and will sidestep the strong evidence of social determinants of health, as described by Crawshaw: 'the placing of responsibility with the individual represents a cynical preparation for the failure of social policy' (Crawshaw 2013: 635).

Implication for practice 4.3
Using the four Ps of the marketing mix, explain how digital technology can enhance health promotion practice.

Summary conclusion

The most prevalent chronic conditions in the affluent North are cancer, cardiovascular diseases, obstructive lung diseases and diabetes, as well as issues relating to mental health and sexual health. Behavioural factors are the leading causes of chronic health conditions and injuries worldwide, with an associated increase of healthcare costs (CSDH 2008). Unhealthy lifestyles or habits include smoking, physical inactivity, excessive alcohol consumption and high calorie intake, leading to obesity, high blood pressure, high cholesterol levels. Many of these non-communicable diseases are preventable, and many health risk factors are modifiable. Targeting people with higher risks is more cost-effective. However, raising awareness and knowledge and changing attitudes are often insufficient to improve health outcomes. Population-based health promotion activities in general are ineffective, as compliance with health behaviour-change messages can be difficult for some. Laverack (2017) asserted that the behaviour approach can, at best, support policy to promote health and, at worst, contribute to inequality in society. Behaviour approaches simply don't impact on the broader conditions that influence health. He suggested that a multipronged approach – a behaviour approach, together with an empowerment approach and a strong policy framework that create a supportive environment – would be more effective. The use of sophisticated innovative and interactive digital technology health promotion programmes might be designed to fit the purpose. However, people do not always act as 'rationally' as professionals would expect. Fundamentally, people do not resist change, but they do resist being changed (Laverack 2017). 'Compliance' is not only determined by a person's intention, motivation and ability to change; it also depends on external social, economic and environmental factors that influence their decision-making processes.

Behaviour theories and models can help to predict and explain people's behaviour, but they have limited success in achieving better health outcomes, or even giving measures of effectiveness. For interventions to succeed, the causal risk factors for the target behaviour need to be clear, and the potential for interventions to reduce the risk needs to be high. Theoretical efficacy needs to be sound. The social and environmental context and the transferability of the programme also need to be considered, as do the meaning and context of people's behaviour practice. Information provision and empowerment approaches can seem simplistic and unrealistic. Other means and government commitment are necessary for health improvement (CSDH 2008).

The WHO (CSDH 2008) provided some guidelines for successful behavioural interventions:

- strong leadership, ownership and commitment
- multi-pronged interventions
- multi-level interventions
- timing is crucial
- adequate resources
- thorough assessment of the (dis)incentives and cues for action.

Effective intervention needs a thorough analysis of the health issue, proper planning strategies and the involvement of all stakeholders. Monitoring and evaluation are essential (CSDH 2008). The success of individualistic behavioural and lifestyle approaches is limited, even with the development of innovative technology. Healthy public policy and the provision of a supportive and enabling environment are important in health promotion. Thus, tackling the social, economic and environmental determinants of health, as well as the co-ordination of all stakeholders, is needed, particularly including the population whom we are working with: a bottom-up empowerment approach. The vast amount of personal and service data collected through digital technologies is also useful for public health service planning. We will look at the management of public health services and the Big Data phenomenon, and the issue of health inequalities, in the next two chapters.

5

Big Data and Public Health Management

Key points

- To set out the public health issues in recent years.
- To discuss the management of public health and the public health workforce in the digital age.
- To discuss the use of digital technology in the management of public health issues.
- To explore the impact of Big Data.
- To consider public health research and surveillance in the Big Data environment.
- To discuss privacy, security and confidentiality, cyberbullying and ethical perspectives.

Introduction

We have seen the rapid development of technologies in the Global North. The Global South is also fast catching up. Electronic and mobile health initiatives are increasingly used in healthcare delivery in many countries (WHO 2011a; Javitt 2014). The development of digital technologies can contribute to health promotion, and individual and community empowerment. They can support comprehensive health data management systems through the development of digital platforms where health data can be shared among relevant professionals. This can improve accessibility of health information, providing efficient and effective services, improving health outcomes. A central focus of this chapter is the fact that advanced digital technologies produce Big Data. This is new territory as compared with twenty years ago. The surveillance abilities of digital technologies mean that large amounts of personal data can be collected, monitored, analysed and reused. This would impact on consumers and citizens in a commercial environment where details of consumer behaviours are collected and used for commercial gain. It would also impact on professionals at the macro level in the management of public health issues, and health practitioners at the micro level, working to improve health outcomes.

As information access, information sharing and the use of tracking devices become more common, the sensitivity and complexity of vast amounts of personal and health data need examination (Lupton 2015c; WHO 2011a). Data storage and retrieval access, privacy and data security are increasingly major issues (WHO 2011a; Lupton 2015c) as can be seen in the recent (May 2017) cyberattack on the UK's NHS, when many health service computers were locked by a ransomware program. There are also risks in the use of social media for our privacy – for example, to do with confidentiality, ownership issues, cyberbullying (Lafferty 2013). This can be seen in the recent use of Facebook personal data by Cambridge Analytica. The ownership and reuse of readily available data have become a concern, ethically and politically.

Previous chapters reviewed the development of digital technology in the past decade, setting out the main theoretical and practical issues relating to the use of technology. This chapter looks more specifically at the management of public health in this digitized environment, the impact of this complex web of information and knowledge on the global and globalized populations – the Big Data phenomenon in a connected world. It will explore the collection of health data and their management, the use of data for health surveillance and monitoring, providing evidence-based practice for health service planning and health needs assessment, and the implications of Big Data. The education and training needs for health promotion practitioners will also be discussed, reflecting on skills and competencies as described by the *Public Health Skills and Knowledge Framework* (PHE 2016b), and internationally by the IUHPE's *Core Competencies and Professional Standards for Health Promotion* (IUHPE 2016).

Public health in the last two decades

According to the WHO (2017c) Public Health report, health and life expectancy have improved everywhere. Over the past ten year period (2007–17), the number of people dying from HIV and malaria fell by 50 per cent; TB and infant death were also dramatically reduced. However, in the twenty-first century, the pressures from ageing, rapid urbanization, and global marketing of unhealthy products have all led to an increase of chronic non-communicable disease overtaking infectious disease as the leading killer worldwide. Chronic non-communicable diseases, such as heart disease, diabetes, cancer and chronic respiratory diseases, which were once only linked to affluent countries, are now global. People in poverty suffer most. Within the European region, we are on target to achieve Health 2020 in reducing premature death from cardiovascular diseases, cancer, diabetes and respiratory diseases (WHO 2015). Most improvements in this region are from countries with the highest premature mortality. Alcohol consumption, tobacco use, unhealthy diet, obesity and physical inactivity are important issues. Mental health – for example, depression, healthy ageing, dementia, malnutrition to obesity, road injury, younger disabled people, and women and children suffering from violence have also become important issues in the last ten years.

The WHO (2017c) report stated that no country has managed to turn around its obesity epidemic among all age groups. The WHO proposed a universal coverage for health. It sees this as the ultimate expression of fairness, ensuring no one is left behind (2017c). In 2015, at least half of the world's population did not have full coverage of essential health services. Sustainable Development Goal 3 (SDG3 – about good health and wellbeing for people, ensuring healthy lives and promoting wellbeing for all at all ages, one of the seventeen SDGs set by the United Nations in 2015) aims to achieve universal health coverage 'to ensure that every individual and community, irrespective of their circumstances, should receive the health services they need without risking financial hardship' (WHO 2017a: 13). Universal health coverage also helps with achieving other health-related SDGs, such as SDG 1 (no poverty), SDG 4 (quality education), SDG 5 (gender equality), SDG 16 (inclusive societies) and SDG 8 (inclusive economic growth and decent jobs). Equity is key to the SDGs, and fairness in access to care is an ethical imperative.

Managing public health and the public health workforce

Using England as an example to illustrate public health responses, the purpose of this section is to highlight some of the issues that *all* public health functions may face in a globalized, digitized world. It is not intended to be a full, cross-national comparison of public health, which would be beyond the scope or focus of this book. Readers from other countries will need to reflect on their own country and their own public health circumstances. In England, public health indicators have followed past trajectories over the period 2009–15. According to Davies et al. (2016), from QualityWatch, there is a reduction in the number of people who had set a quit date to stop smoking with the NHS stop-smoking services, but there was an increase of sexually transmitted infection (STI) and alcohol-related hospital admissions. Uptake of Long Acting Reversible Contraception, genital warts prevalence, drug treatment waiting time, smoking in pregnancy and childhood obesity among 4- to 5-year-olds are improving. There are also areas where there are promising signs – e.g., smoking prevalence, teenage pregnancy, late-diagnosis HIV, completion of substance misuse treatment, and MMR uptake. Some (e.g. the proportion of smokers who actually quit and the number of substance misusers in treatment) are unclear and some (e.g. childhood obesity among 10- to 11-year-olds and childhood immunization) seem to have stayed the same. Trends have been variable across the country, with the most socioeconomically deprived areas disproportionately affected by worsening trends in STI rates, compared to the national average. But more deprived areas have improved in teenage pregnancy rates.

In England, Public Health moved to local authority control in 2013. This was seen as a welcome reorganization. It demonstrated the government's recognition of the importance of social, environmental and economic factors that influence health. Public health practitioners are now well placed to work with other departments within local councils and their local communities. However, the structure of the system is rather complex! Some public health functions, such as immunization and screening programmes, along with some specialist services such as prison health and sexual assault referral services, remain with the Health Service. There was a further fragmentation of public health services after the Health and Social Care Act 2012, with a detrimental effect on service availability and patient care (House of Commons Health Committee 2016). It was also reported by the Commons Select Committee on Public Health post-2013 that data sharing, for example, of local screening and immunization rates, was restricted. In this digital age, it is surprising and disappointing that health data on the population – e.g. population healthcare data and operational data about the services public health specialists commissioned, can only be accessed centrally within NHS Digital by the public health workforce.

Under the Health Act 2007, Health and Wellbeing boards within local authorities have the responsibility to assess and develop a Joint Strategic Needs Assessment and Joint Health and Wellbeing Strategy to improve the health and wellbeing of the local population and reduce inequality for all ages (Department of Health 2013a). The secondary uses of data can help in the assessment of needs. However, the link between systems was cancelled due to data security concerns. With the restriction of health data access, the public health workforce is unable to access health information to do their job. This has become a barrier for public health practitioners working locally to plan services to meet local needs. Similarly, the fragmentation of the public health protection function is also problematic, e.g. in the sharing of and access to data on health protection incidents, and engaging with other NHS services, as well as understanding the role and responsibilities of each organization (House of Commons Health Committee 2016).

The public health workforce with a role in improving the health of their population is composed of a range of different professionals – e.g. health visitors and school nurses, public health consultants, public health managers, environmental health professionals, as well as public health scientists. Unfortunately, the public health dataset has not been implemented and there are no direct comparable data to assess how the workforce is changing over time. Health visitors (public health nursing) and those with a specific health-related qualification are subject to their statutory professional regulation. Interestingly, non-statutory public health workers are the second-largest group of public health professionals. They are covered by voluntary registration, but not governed by legislation. Statutory regulation is there to ensure public safety and confidence. It is disappointing that government has not taken this forward into policy. The public health workforce includes many without health-related professional status – such as health trainers, health promotion specialists working at ground level; there seems to be no mention of these important groups. They are not acknowledged as having a place within the public health workforce. This is not a new finding that strategies in health and social care fail to address, consult or prioritize face-to-face workers who are crucial to the delivery of services (Beresford et al. 2011).

All of this is happening while digital technology is a rapidly growing area in public health. With cuts in public health budgets (HM Government 2015; HM Treasury 2015; PHPSU 2015; Davies et al. 2016), the funding for training of public health practitioners and for the training of staff in the use of new technologies is limited. Education and training are needed to ensure their need for skills and competencies – as described by the *Public Health Skills and Knowledge Framework* (PHE 2016b), and internationally by the IUHPE's *Core Competencies and Professional Standards for Health Promotion* (IUHPE 2016) – is met in addressing public health issues.

The House of Commons Health Committee report (2016) agreed some areas are doing well in public health, incorporating health into their policy planning, whereas others need improvement. From a social model of health and social determinants point of view, there are advantages in public health operating within local government, where there is potential for more whole-system working relationships across departments. However, there is a concern that the emphasis on prevention in the *NHS Five Year Forward View* (NHS 2014) will have been weakened with public health no longer being in the remit of the NHS. This is compounded by the fragmentation of service delivery, and inefficient IT systems denying staff access to information to do their job. Variations in performance between local authorities, and unclear accountabilities, tension between politics and evidence, boundary issues and fragmentation, workforce issues and poor access to data and information are barriers for improving health outcomes. It is important that health considerations are taken into account in all policies. To manage public health issues efficiently and effectively, and to improve health outcomes, data collection needs to be strengthened and new health-monitoring approaches explored (WHO 2015). Political attention to combatting public health issues is important and is a powerful way to improve longevity and healthy life expectancy.

Reflection 5.1

If you have experience as a health professional, how well organized is your public health management system in your area of practice? How has technology improved the public health functioning, and improved health outcomes, for the population you serve? What challenges do you face, if any?

The use of digital technology in the management of public health services

Health information technology has been a major part of the UK NHS technology reform since the first National Information Technology Strategy for the NHS (NHS Management Executive 1992) and the launch of the UK National Programme for Information Technology (NPfIT) in 1998. The programme was set up in 2002, and replaced by Connecting for Health in 2005. This IT programme was successful in developing email systems for staff to exchange information, e-prescribing and a diagnostic imaging system, scheduling and booking of consultations, and electronic health records allowing professionals instant access to patient health history, e.g. during emergency consultation. It was believed that these developments would improve the quality of services and reduce the cost of healthcare. Unfortunately, overall implementation was unsuccessful and led to closure of the programme in 2011 (Waterson 2014; Honeyman et al. 2016).

In 2012, a *Digital Strategy Report* (Department of Health 2012a: 6) was published, making advanced technology 'a major priority', 'launching a health information revolution that put patients in control of their own health and care information making health services convenient, accessible and efficient'. The then Secretary of State for Health, Jeremy Hunt, in 2013 challenged the NHS to 'go paperless' by 2018 (Hunt 2013). The publication of the *NHS Five Year Forward View* followed (NHS 2014), and was subsequently extended to 2020. The National Information Board was then set up to lead and support the digitization of the health and care system. The Scottish government is also committed to a world-class digital service in its 2020 vision report (Scottish Government 2013), allowing instant access to information, anytime, anywhere, and promoting a cultural acceptance of digital healthcare services. The transformation of health and social care is about empowering everyone to live longer and healthier. Health promoting services need interconnectedness for fast and effective service provision, such as emergency services, and routine or chronic illness management.

Waterson (2014) agreed with the need for a new Health Information System. The Department of Health report *The Power of Information* (Department of Health 2012b) restated the original goals of NPfIT and the ten-year 'Information Strategy' for the health and care system. However, there was no plan for achieving it (Waterson 2014). There is also concern that history is repeating itself – e.g. recognizing that developments have to be local to meet local needs, establishing standards for interoperability and not following the one-size-fits-all approach, but at the same time suggesting that the new system should be standardized for aggregated and demographic comparisons across the whole of the NHS (Waterson 2014).

The development of healthcare information technology was perceived as improving information exchange, and increasing consistency between different services as well as economic efficiency. For example, both the UK and the USA spend large sums of money on healthcare informatics, such as electronic health records. However, healthcare information systems are complex. Examples of system failure have occurred both in the UK (2006) and in the USA (2007) (Johnson 2010). Problems arise when system failures occur. The increasing use of ICT can transform health systems (Kwankam 2012). The International Society for Telemedicine and eHealth proposed a national eHealth infrastructure, which includes a National eHealth council – providing policy advice to the government and overseeing eHealth, and consisting of professional health workers – an eHealth steering committee and an eHealth centre of excellence, supported by a national eHealth society and a forum for health professionals to exchange ideas and share knowledge (Kwankam 2012). However, for progress to be made, ICT needs to be woven into the fabric of the health system at policy and practice level (UN 2011).

In the UK as a whole, there has been technological progress in primary care; however, the use of modern technology in the acute, community and mental health sectors has been slow (Honeyman et al. 2016; Wachter 2016). There is a general agreement that digital technology has the potential to modernize and transform healthcare. However, cost savings from digitization in healthcare require up-front investment and time for development and delivery. Also, a focus on costs may look to get the same levels of care within a reduced budget (a saving to accountancy) rather than better care for the same budget (a benefit to patients). In the age of austerity, and with healthcare systems being constantly under pressure, the UK government has not been clear on how funding will be provided for such large-scale IT reform (Waterson 2014; Honeyman et al. 2016; Wachter 2016). The priorities and timescales are also unclear. The Wachter review (2016) emphasized the use of innovative technology in healthcare during this 'information revolution' period. However, IT systems need to be maintained and upgraded constantly. When system failure occurs, as seen in 2016 when a ransom malware demanded payment for NHS computer use, it emphasizes the importance of staff training in coping with IT failure and the use of technology at work. Data security is also important. Countries need to learn from each other. Users of technology – all stakeholders and patients – will also need to be involved (Honeyman et al. 2016).

Next Steps on the NHS Five Year Forward View in England (NHS 2017) is built on the recommendations of the Wachter review (2016). It extensively discussed incentivizing and supporting healthier behaviour, local democratic leadership, working with local authorities, helping people to stay in employment, etc. It also talked about the NHS as a social movement. In harnessing technology and innovation, the document discussed the government's ambition to simplify patients' access to care in the appropriate location; to help people take a more active role in their own health; to digitize hospitals – for example, by making it easier for patients to access urgent care online or by phone, NHS 111 online (triage services) enables patients to enter their symptoms and receive tailored advice or a call-back; to facilitate use of NHS health apps and the health and care website (NHS.UK), e-prescription services, and viewing one's own record; to improve the online appointment booking process; to make patients' medical information available to the right clinicians wherever they are; to make WiFi free in GP surgeries.

While controlling service costs, eHealth systems have the potential to improve public health outcomes. Electronic applications and platforms can help improve health surveillance and health system management for health education and clinical decision-making processes, to support behavioural changes related to public health priorities and disease management. For example, fully interoperable electronic health records, with the capacity for patients to write into them, is a commitment of the government (NHS 2014). In the UK, all patients have been able to see their summary care record since April 2015, as is the case with all citizens in the European Union. An earlier initiative wasn't successful as there was no demand for it, and its functionality aligned poorly with patient's self-management practice (Coulter and Mearns 2016). In a study by Shah et al. (2015), patients were positive towards viewing their own records as being convenient, useful, usable and flexible, although the provision is limited and the number of patients requesting to see their records is small. Regardless of issues of cost-effectiveness, patients are more in control of their own healthcare. They also have a better understanding of their own health status, are better prepared for their consultation and better able to understand their clinical management. In contrast with previous concerns on confidentiality and data accuracy of personal health information, there were no concerns about these among participants in this particular research.

A review from Piette et al. (2012) on chronic ill health management, cost-effectiveness of eHealth approaches and the impact of eHealth showed that electronic medical records are widely used in Denmark, the Netherlands, Sweden and the UK, but less so in the US. Electronic medical record systems are also available in large specialist hospitals in low- and middle-income countries. The use of picture archiving and communication systems is rapidly increasing in low- and middle-income countries. However, there is more evidence of benefits for tools that support clinical decisions and laboratory information systems than for those that support picture archiving and communication systems. The study also showed that disease surveillance systems have been implemented successfully in some low- and middle-income countries. There are also documented notable impacts on health system efficiency, for example in Brazil. However, information on health outcomes is generally lacking.

Managing long-term conditions is one of the most important challenges for any health service. In the UK, long-term conditions took up 50% of GP appointments, 64% of hospital outpatient appointments, and 70% of inpatient bed days, accounting for 70% of healthcare expenditure (Department of Health 2012c). A proactive system in managing this area of healthcare is important both for cost-effectiveness and for improving health outcomes. Computer programmes and apps can help support the co-produced care planning processes whereby patients and care professionals work together to manage chronic conditions. Individuals at risk can be targeted and benefit from the use of Big Data and predictive algorithms, through predictive risk analysis. Online real-time feedback is also becoming more popular. Programmes such as 'Patient Opinion' or 'I want great care' can provide data on patients' experience and improve quality of care. Local community groups and services can also be incorporated into the electronic health directories to facilitate signposting and referral. However, this type of bottom-up approach is rare (Coulter and Mearns 2016).

The fundamental benefit of telemedicine is in the improvement of access to healthcare. The progress is much slower in low- and middle-income countries than in developed countries. There are some examples of telemedicine in telecommunications and education for health professionals needing advice and clinical management of difficult cases, e.g. via emails and video links. Some eHealth interventions, such as automated telephone monitoring and self-care support calls, have been shown to improve some outcomes of chronic disease management, for example in glycaemia and blood pressure control. However, more information on the impacts of these eHealth interventions on outcomes and costs in low-resource settings is needed (Piette et al. 2012). Good data quality and good health information systems are important to address health challenges and improve health service delivery

(Braa et al. 2012). A review by Wootton et al. (2012) studying seven well-established telemedicine networks in low- and middle-income countries showed that these networks provide reasonable evidence of improving access to care in the developing world. However, the scientific framework, such as study design and evaluation of parameters – e.g. effectiveness – is weak. Collaboration between networks may help overcome resource shortages and improve sustainability. Stronger evidence and better evaluation of telemedicine networks is needed.

Implication for practice 5.1

How might you get feedback from your clients on health promotion campaigns? How helpful might digital technology be for you in getting feedback from clients on the service you provide? If you have experience of health promotion practice, is getting feedback on your service a norm in your practice?

Managing challenges – cyberbullying

The fast progression of digital technologies has brought many opportunities. However, there are also many challenges. For example, with the increased use of computers, tablets and smartphones, screen time has become an issue over the past few years, with smartphone apps that can inform you of your daily screen time. We have discussed the use of digital technology in chapter 2 relating to, for example, young people and obesity and physical inactivity. Key messages from the Royal College of Paediatric and Child Health (RCPCH 2018) stated that the evidence base for negative effect of prolonged screen time is contested. It produced recommendations for health professionals and families on screen time management in 2019.

One particular challenge in managing internet use among young people is in the area of cyberbullying. Cyberbullying has become a public health problem worldwide. With the commercialization and increased use of internet and social media, as with many systems, there is a risk of abuse by people using it. Arguably, bullying is a safeguarding issue; however, safeguarding itself is also a public health issue. Policies and regulations need to be in place to ensure the safety of users. Although cyberbullying may be less prevalent than traditional bullying, it is a global phenomenon and has a detrimental effect on young people's mental health (Akar 2017; Tozun and Babaoglu 2017).

In a study on paediatric emergency department attendees, Roberts et al. (2016) found that cyberbullying prevalence is the same as traditional bullying, cyberbullying victims have more suicidal ideation, and experience more physical, sexual and emotional abuse and a higher admission rate, especially among females. Bullying is defined as repeated acts of violence towards victims, on the basis of a power imbalance. Cyberbullying is deliberate and repeated damage to someone using digital technologies. While the act of cyberbullying is more common among boys, girls are reported as more likely to be the victims. Ethnicity, gender and sexuality other than heterosexuality can also be risk factors (Tozun and Babaoglu 2017). Cyberbullying is a mental health as well as social health issue, leading to problems such as depression, loneliness, suicidal tendencies, lower academic achievement, isolation, anxiety, low self-esteem and relationship problems (Lee et al. 2013; Roberts et al. 2016; Akar 2017; Tozun and Babaoglu 2017). Akar (2017) found that the causes and consequences of cyberbullying are similar to those of bullying. Family and schools are best placed to prevent cyberbullying and to support victims. Increasing the awareness at individual, institutional and societal levels is needed. Interventions such as technical web protection – e.g. blocking, password changing – online psychological therapy, counselling, and social and communication skills development are useful. The cyberbully also needs help – e.g. in managing anger or stress (Akar 2017).

Technology is the driving force in globalization. Countries such as South Africa, Nigeria and Kenya are emerging economies (Ephraim 2013) where social media are increasingly becoming important interpersonal communication tools, particularly for young people. Cyberbullying and cyberviolence were already experienced by many, particularly girls and women, and many incidents were unreported and undocumented. South Africa has the highest prevalence of cyberbullying among African countries, Morocco ranked 7th and Egypt 21st in 2012 (Ephraim 2013). The lack of legislation, policy or any mechanisms to address cybercrime incidents is a concern. Technologies such as the mobile phone have given young people a new kind of freedom (Ephraim 2013). Ephraim called for a culture-centred approach to using social media in which the rights and dignities of others are respected regardless of age, gender, race, social status or sexual orientation. Young people should learn to uphold ethical and moral standards and respect for cultural norms and values, and to become responsible users of social networks. Ground rules should be set as guides. Family, school, government agencies, religious organizations, mass media, all have a role to play in the use of culture-centred approaches (Ephraim 2013). However, the lack of technical knowledge and awareness of parents in these countries could be a challenge. Responsibility for the operational gaps in social media lie with the government, as well as the privacy and data security measures of the service provider. Some legislation has been approved in countries such as South Africa. Cybercrime prevention centres and websites have been established to protect children and women. However, countries with older regulations approved before the digital revolution need to keep their legislation up to date (Ephraim 2013).

Cyberbullying exposes ethical issues. Linking to the discussion of health promotion ethics in chapter 3, according to a deontological, duty-based, ethical position proposed by Kant, we have a duty to act in accordance with certain universal moral rules. What is right is independent of any situation. What is wrong will always be wrong, regardless of consequences. However, according to Utilitarian ethics from Bentham and Mill, right or wrong depends on the consequences – a consequential ethics, focusing on achieving the greatest collective benefits. If the choices made affect more people than an individual, intervention may be necessary for the greater good – e.g. a smoking ban. However, with the complexity of Big Data, it is problematic to determine the relative position. Due to the complexity of dataset linkages, informed consent can be rather unclear. There may be rules regarding privacy and data sharing – however, the actual situation is rather difficult to control. Autonomy can't always be guaranteed. There is also the issue of professionalism in the use of social media – e.g. regarding posting unacceptable images or unprofessional behaviour online. Social media are like a mirror: they can reflect the best and worst aspects of the content placed before them for all to see (Greysen et al. 2010).

A study by Harrison (2016) found that, from a deontological perspective, there was a perceived absence of clear rules online among young people, leading to an increased sense of freedom.

Internet anonymity enabled them to bypass their ordinary duties, and made them more likely to do things that they would not normally do offline. Anonymity also diminishes accountability and reduces sensitivity towards victims. Many participants in his study acknowledged that there are people they knew who acted differently online, adopting a different internet lifestyle and identity. Many of his participants acknowledged that they did not read terms and conditions on the internet as they were not issued by a person and there was nobody enforcing them. With the scale of the internet, young people doubt whether rules could ever be enforced, particularly as the internet is often used when young people are on their own.

From a Utilitarian perspective, features on the internet also make utilitarian principles challenging. The internet is impersonal and faceless. Consequences of online communications are hard to determine. Hence, if direct consequences are not seen, it is less likely that guilt will be felt when someone is hurt. From a Virtue Ethics perspective, the absence of certain virtues – such as care, self-discipline, compassion, humility, trust – appears to allow the bully to bully others. The decision whether to bully or not depends on the quality of the person. People should take responsibility for themselves. Harrison (2016) also found that some features on the internet inhibit bullying – e.g., everyone can see what you write. Written communications can also inhibit, as written messages are permanent compared to oral communication. From this study, Harrison felt that a moral theory, as in Virtue Ethics, that prioritizes human character could be used complementarily to duties-based deontological or consequential ethics when finding solutions for cyberbullying. While a deontological approach might continue to be helpful to set rules and guidance governing online conduct, and a Utilitarian one could draw greater attention to harmful consequences, a Virtue Ethical perspective would help with the formation of wise and virtuous online citizens.

Reflection 5.2

What forms of cyberbullying could exist relating to your work as a health promotion professional – emails? Twitter? Other social media? Text messaging? Between colleagues? Between professionals and clients? Do you think it's easier for one person to bully another on the internet because you don't see the other person face to face? How can we prevent cyberbullying happening?

The Big Data phenomenon

Of all of the changes brought about by the increase in digital usage, none is more significant than the Big Data phenomenon. The mathematics of connectedness have created this unforeseen and unexpected result. According to Kemp (2018), more than two-thirds of the world's inhabitants in 2017 had a mobile phone, and more than half of the handsets in use were smart devices. On average, internet users spend 6 hours each day using internet-powered devices and services. Some regions, such as Central Africa and Southern Asia, have a low penetration rate, but these are also seeing the fastest growth in internet adoption. Mobile phones see the highest web traffic, e.g. 95.1 per cent of Facebook users access the platform via their mobile phone or tablets. Facebook still dominates the global social landscape, with YouTube, WhatsApp, Facebook Messenger and WeChat following. WhatsApp has the strongest geographic position and is the top messenger app in 128 countries around the world. There are also many social media users joining Facebook who are aged 65 and above. However, the number of women using Facebook across Central Africa, the Middle East and Southern China is still comparatively low. Mobile connection speeds are getting faster all over the world, with Norway, Malta, the Netherlands, Singapore, the UAE and Iceland enjoying the fastest connection speeds, and India and Indonesia the slowest. Ecommerce also grew rapidly, with 45 per cent of all internet users using it to buy goods online (Kemp 2018).

The internet has radically changed the way people access information and make decisions about their lives. We communicate via the internet, sharing information freely about ourselves on social media intentionally, via personal communications such as email and social networking sites, or exchanging information about our medical conditions with healthcare professionals. We also share information unintentionally about ourselves via e-commerce transactions, search engines, mobile phone apps, etc. These data can be mined, analysed, repackaged and repurposed as part of data assemblage, whereby data are constantly disassembled and reassembled to provide insights into our health/commercial behaviour for secondary uses (Kitchin and Lauriault 2014). We live in a panopticon world, under surveillance continuously through the use of our technological devices, a concept originated by Foucault. Whenever we use technology, our information is gathered, analysed through data mining technology, repackaged and commodified. The panoptical gaze in a surveillance society has power over us, and we voluntarily and willingly become self-managers of our own health (Lupton 2012).

When we search for something on the internet, very quickly we will see advertisements in our browser about our searches. It can be puzzling that our brief glance at a product in an online store suddenly becomes an embedded advert in our Facebook browsing session. The pizza joke below, although a joke about internet use, does illustrate how much we are under surveillance, how much of our personal data are floating around and used, with huge implications for issues such as privacy and confidentiality, and with data security and ethics concerns.

Joke for the Era of Big Data *(This joke is pretty ubiquitous across the internet.)*

Hello! Is this Gordon's Pizza?
No sir, it's Google's Pizza.
Did I dial the wrong number?
No sir, Google bought the pizza store.
Oh, alright – then I'd like to place an order please.
Okay sir, do you want the usual?
The usual? You know what my usual is?
According to the caller ID, the last 15 times you've ordered a 12-slice with double-cheese, sausage, and thick crust.
Okay – that's what I want this time too.
May I suggest that this time you order an 8-slice with ricotta, arugula, and tomato instead?
No, I hate vegetables.
But your cholesterol is not good.
How do you know?
Through the subscribers' guide. We have the results of your blood tests for the last 7 years.
Maybe so, but I don't want the pizza you suggest – I already take medicine for high cholesterol.
But you haven't taken the medicine regularly. 4 months ago you purchased from Drugsale Network a box of only 30 tablets.
I bought more from another drugstore.
It's not showing on your credit card sir.
I paid in cash.
But according to your bank statement you did not withdraw that much cash.
I have another source of cash.

This is not showing on your last tax form, unless you got it from an undeclared income source.

To HELL With Ur Pizza . . . !! I'm sick of Google, Facebook, Twitter, and WhatsApp. I'm going to an island without internet, where there's no cellphone network, and no one to spy on me . . .

I understand sir, but you'll need to renew your PASSPORT . . . it expired 5 weeks ago.

Big Data is about capturing, storing, sharing, evaluating and acting upon information that people and devices have created and distributed via computer-based technologies and networks (Herschel and Miori 2017). It is about the accumulation of large amounts of digital data from a wide range of electronic sources at high velocity (Barrett et al. 2013). With the improvement of telecommunication technology and high-speed transmission of data globally, there is an increase in volume, variety, velocity and veracity, as well as variability and complexity, of data (Herschel and Miori 2017). Organizational computers were once the main creators of data. New social, personal digital communications, such as video sharing, social media and location services, have now accelerated the growth of data. They provide commercial opportunities with an understanding and prediction of consumer behaviour. The media, traditional or internet, are importance sources of information for many; they can also be used for reporting of health and related events, providing early warning signs for disease outbreaks. Medicine 2.0 / Health 2.0 is about the use of Web 2.0 tools by healthcare actors, with the active participation of individuals in their healthcare. Increased internet use has also enabled populations' participation in healthcare management.

Reflection 5.3

Have you ever wondered how your computer seems to know what you want to buy, what you want to do? How worried are you, for example, when you give your bank details and pay for your goods online? What measures, if any, have you put in place to protect your privacy, and confidentiality of your personal details?

Internet public health research and surveillance

In the public health arena, most internet research is about surveillance and monitoring of health behaviour (Hill et al. 2013). Big datasets generated from digital technology can be used to identify risks and develop public health and health promotion strategies. Online data about patterns of diseases can be collected and used in 'Infodemiology' and 'infoveillance', e.g. queries and search terms can be tracked and analysed to monitor diseases such as influenza (Lupton 2012). Risks can be assessed, and interventions developed. Through online crowd surveillance, internet data can be collected, mined and repackaged by academics, business and government, via surveillance systems, providing insights into health/commercial behaviour (Hill et al. 2013). The large 'crowd' group of internet users can provide population-level information. The Quantified Self, as discussed by Barrett et al. (2013), refers to self-monitoring of one's own health and behaviour. A person's body can become a set of empirical measurements and digital data (Lupton 2015b). Self-surveillance data from the Quantified Self – such as physical activity information from Fitbit, diet, sleep quality, drug adherence – can be accumulated and aggregated to a population level, becoming a Quantified Community, and be very useful for surveillance. Electronic health records and self-monitoring health apps also provide rich and detailed data about people over longer periods of time, more rich and robust than traditional epidemiological studies (Barrett et al. 2013; Hill et al. 2013).

Digital disease surveillance is a useful method, complementary to traditional epidemiology and disease monitoring approaches (Hswen et al. 2017; Schwind et al. 2017). Population-level information gathered via the internet reflects the public's health concerns (Prier et al. 2011; Hill et al. 2013; Karami et al. 2018). Social media, such as Twitter, and search engines can provide a platform for people to broadcast information and thoughts about their daily lives, ranging from politics to earthquake monitoring. They can reflect opinions and concerns from a wide population and provide fast and cheap updates about real-world events (Dredze 2012) – for example, in natural disaster management in emergencies and in non-emergency health-related issues such as predicting flu epidemics using 'Flu Near You' (Dredze 2012); in mental health; for clarifying medical misconceptions; for risk assessment in CHD, or in diabetes and related issues (Karami et al. 2018), or regarding tobacco use (Prier et al. 2011). Crowdsourcing as a method in participatory public health research is particularly useful for monitoring the spread of infectious diseases in real time. Crowdsourced health research studies can also complement and support traditional clinical trials (Swan 2012; Barrett et al. 2013). These can be professionally led, such as PatientsLikeMe, or participant-led, such as Quantified Self. The participants are recruited via internet-based techniques, to become the drivers of their own health (Swan 2012).

Big Data can help in assessing the health needs of a given population, assisting in the statutory Joint Strategy Needs Assessment and the Joint Health and Wellbeing Strategy. Data mining technologies can make unstructured data accessible, timely and meaningful (Barrett et al. 2013). With analytics and data mining, Big Data provides opportunities for understanding and predicting consumer behaviour. Linking to people's electronic health records, it can be a useful way to determine effective interventions and targeted health promotion (Hill et al. 2013). Using Thermia, an online and mobile education tool, Hswen et al. (2017) found that sourcing data from online tools can help predict influenza outbreaks a month earlier than traditional National Health and Family Planning Commission influenza surveillance systems. They found that data sourcing from the internet is potentially more consistent and less subject to human error. However, the accuracy also depends on who uses the app and how. Social media research is particularly useful for filling in information gaps which traditional public health research can't cover – for example, on weight loss, smoking cessation or health promoting physical activity programmes, as these depend on people outside the clinical setting, demonstrating the potential of using internet research for self-management and health promotion interventions (Dredze 2012).

There are also non-health data on the environment, for example climate, pollution levels, traffic patterns, water quality, land use, socioeconomic data, crime data, social networks, etc. These all feed into Big Data, particularly in terms of social, economic and environmental determinants of health. Geographical information gives the social and environmental context of self-tracking data, e.g. Smartphone can provide contextual information such as symptoms, perceived triggers and activity in individuals with asthma; and Asthmapolis can track the time and location of inhaler use by communicating with smartphones. Aggregated data can identify local asthma hotspots within a region, and be combined with environmental data giving information on environmental factors influencing the condition. Data-driven approaches can assist individual and community-level disease management (Barrett et al. 2013).

Rapid internet growth can enable collection of large volumes of health-related data that are cheaper, richer in content and faster. Crowdsourcing of data is useful for individuals, for researchers and for commercial applications. It has the potential for health-related research, improving the quality, cost and speed of a research project (Barrett et al. 2013; Hill et al. 2013; Yank et al. 2017), for example in problem solving, data processing, surveillance/monitoring, and surveying of public-health-related issues (Ranard et al. 2013). However, data accuracy is debatable – e.g. in the representation and generalization of research participants, as participants are self-selected and data are self-reported (Swan 2012; Yank 2017). In an American study, Yank (2017) found that crowdsourced participants for health research are younger, and more likely to be white with higher levels of educational attainment. Crowdsourced research has the potential to expand citizen participation, but also to exacerbate health disparities and magnify inclusion and exclusion effects. Thus, there is a need to be careful and aware of the issues of sampling for research using crowdsourcing techniques.

In general, public health research is needed to identify risk factors in disease prevention from medical and behavioural approach points of view. Big Data, in this context, is not simply about commercial surveillance. It can be useful for positive health promotion at the population level, as well as offering possibilities for empowerment and choice (Barrett et al. 2013). It can provide beneficial health surveillance, as well as communication tools for health promotion messages ranging from exercise to diet and social support. An asset-based approach to health promotion is about empowerment, building agency in the individual and social capital in the community to bring about social changes (Cross et al. 2017). Social networking sites are popular for health promotion interventions. However, evaluation has not kept pace with implementation, although the number of evaluations is growing. Evaluating the reach, engagement and effectiveness of social media interventions is difficult because of the complexity of accurate measurement. There is also a lack of guidance for programme planners on measuring the effectiveness of interventions. In a systematic review, Lim et al. (2016) found that various methods were used for evaluation. However, barriers exist for accurate measurement. Few studies were able to assess rigorously the uptake or effectiveness of real-world interventions.

The internet is powerful in its searchable content and immediacy, as well as in its scale. However, there are also challenges. The vast amount of non-professional health information on the internet, and the time we spend on it compared to medical professional sources, can lead to misinformation. Administration, analysis and management of such large amounts of data can also be difficult, e.g. in distilling the useful data from such large amounts of unstructured internet data (Barrett et al. 2013). Data can also be incomplete and inaccurate, yet they are rich, easily and continuously available in huge volumes. Data without context may also add to inaccuracy (Hill et al. 2013). Different data collected at different spatial and temporal scales, with incomplete data on electronic health records, can also make analysis challenging (Barrett et al. 2013). Reliable sampling can also be problematic (Hill et al. 2013).

Implication for practice 5.2
How often do you evaluate the service you provide? Is research part of your job? How can digital technology help you in the research process?

Ethics, privacy, security and confidentiality relating to the Big Data environment

Digital technologies are widely used in health promotion and health education. The problems with digital technology include inaccurate and misleading information, lack of investment, and widening disparities, as well as issues relating to privacy and safety (Ren et al. 2017). Security, privacy and confidentiality are major ethical challenges of Big Data for policy makers. We live in the 'end of forgetting' era (Bossewitch and Sinnreich 2013). Once data are uploaded onto the cloud, they are difficult to erase (Lupton 2015b). As commercialization of data happens in the business field – e.g. selling of personal data from wearables to other companies – data security is becoming more of a concern (Lupton 2015b). There is a huge amount of personal data floating about – officially, from our personal health records, hospital data and bank data, and unofficially, from software and hardware, social media such as Facebook, wearable devices, smartphone apps, etc. On one hand, the internet offers potential opportunities for public health interventions and research; on the other, the networked nature of internet science does highlight the vulnerability and sensitivity of data sharing, riddled with ethical challenges without clear consensus on how to manage it (Hunter et al. 2018). There is an assumption that digital technology and the data generated are empirical and powerful, potentially leading to better understanding of our body and greater efficiency in care services; little attention has been given to moral and ethical implications (Lupton 2013b).

As already mentioned, the English NHS health apps library set up in 2013 was found to have poor data security (Huckvale et al. 2015). Huckvale et al.'s findings exposed potential shortcomings of the accreditation approach of health apps. The risk of identity disclosure was significant. The health apps library was withdrawn in 2015, with a new NHS Apps library beta and health apps appraising model launched in April 2017. Two other recent examples of large-scale incidents, also already mentioned (one was the UK NHS 'ransom' incident in 2017, leading to a large-scale shutdown of the health information service system; the other was the worldwide transferring of Facebook personal data via Cambridge Analytica), demonstrated the vulnerability of personal information.

According to Herschel and Miori (2017), Big Data is difficult to manage as it is often incomplete and inaccurate, and yet huge amounts of data are often easily and continuously available. Baig et al. (2015) identified two types of mHealth security issues – one is *system* security, including administrative, physical and technical-level security, and the other is *information* security, including data encryption, data integration, authentications and freshness protection. With sophisticated data linking, data mining and data analysis technology, privacy is invaded without users realizing it. Big Data stakeholders, big organizations, also hold power as they control the collection and utilization of Big Data. The secondary uses of datasets also present problems linking to privacy, confidentiality and identity (Herschel and Miori 2017; Hunter et al. 2018). Researchers and individuals can lose control of how data are manipulated, analysed and used.

From a review on the ethics of Big Data, Mittelstadt and Floridi (2016) identified five ethical themes for Big Data research:

- Informed consent – due to rapid technological development, consent to data use cannot be accurately given due to the complexity and multiple linkage of datasets, e.g. informal data in social media (Mittelstadt and Floridi 2016; Herschel and Miori 2017; Hunter et al. 2018). Consent such as 'click wrap' where you just click 'I agree' is insufficient. Often, people don't read the long terms-and-conditions statement in order to facilitate fast access, unlike in traditional research where participants are given a standard reflection period for withdrawal (Hunter et al. 2018). Under the Declaration of Helsinki, participants have the right to make informed decisions. However, withdrawal from internet research can be difficult to guarantee.
- Privacy, including anonymization, confidentiality and data protection – with data mining and analysing technology, the invasiveness, complexity and linkage of multi-datasets of aggregated data can make privacy very difficult to manage and could lead to group-level harm and discrimination (Mittelstadt and Floridi 2016). Data protection may not be covered in internet-based sources or participant-driven data-based research. Data protection legislation lags behind the potential of these new technologies. It is also difficult for many to grasp the different privacy settings or the terms and conditions policy of social media platforms such as Facebook or Twitter. Identification can be traceable, and anonymity is not always guaranteed (Hunter et al. 2018).
- Ownership is also a complex matter – redistributing and modification of data may be restricted; however, the accessibility of datasets can cause problems.
- Epistemology – because of the amount, opacity and pervasiveness of internet data, and the complexity in analysing internet-aggregated data gathered by computer algorithms, research validity and 'objectivity' can be increasingly difficult to maintain and manage.
- The Big Data Divide, including power and control and the digital divide – the huge volumes of Big Data collected and managed by large organizations also cause difficulties for individuals, researchers and small organizations, who lack access to large

datasets or how data is collected, analysed and used, causing a Big Data divide, as described by Mittelstadt and Floridi (2016). The power dynamic over personal data and information places an ever greater degree of control in the hands of marketers and aggregators (Lupton 2015a). There are imbalances of power and knowledge, and inequalities between data subjects and the organizations who analyse and use the data. New forms of power have emerged in this digital age. Internet empires control the digitized economy (Lupton 2014a).

The interpretation of information depends on the context in which it was collected and the perspective of those giving meaning to it. However, contextual understanding of aggregated data is impossible. Aggregation of large amounts of data obscures the complex methodological decisions and ontological and epistemological assumptions that ground research. The stresses and risks for both participants and researchers are also difficult to manage in internet-based health research. Similarly, standard data management issues such as permission, storage, sharing, security, ownership and dissemination of internet data are beyond the researcher's control. We also need to bear in mind the self-serving interests of social media corporations, and consider the often powerless and uninformed individuals within the social media environment (Hunter et al. 2018).

In a study on security concerns on Android mHealth apps, He et al. (2014) raised serious concerns on the use of unencrypted communication over the internet and the use of third-party hosting and storage services by many health apps, which are not easily fixable. As in Huckvale et al.'s (2015) study, encryption of data and inadequate privacy policy are issues. It is important for mHealth app developers to create a set of security and privacy guidelines that offer a baseline for protection. Health apps developers also need to adapt to the continuously changing landscape of technology (He et al. 2014; Huckvale et al. 2015). Many health apps are provided by commercial organizations, rather than medical providers. They can sit outside the scope of existing legal and professional safeguards (Huckvale et al. 2015). The ready availability of mHealth apps represents a paradigm shift with sensitive data handled by mobile apps, and with shared cloud space storage from mainframe systems located with health service providers. With such rapid developments in media platforms and globalized reach, there is confusion as to which country's data protection legislation applies (Hunter et al. 2018).

Data protection from commercial arenas may also not be as stringent as legislation such as the Health Insurance Portability and Accountability Act (HIPAA) 1996 in the USA (US Congressional Committee 1996), the Federal Trade Commission Act (Federal Trade Commission 2006), the Children's Online Privacy Protection Act 1998 (COPPA 1998) or, in Europe, the Data Protection Act / EU General Data Protection Regulation (GDPR 2018). With the new GDPR, researchers will need to provide a clear account of and justification for the good that their research can offer, and the rights of an individual will also need to be clear (Hunter et al. 2018). However, even with such legislation, there are gaps in assuring individual privacy. It is difficult for organizations to interpret legislation (Bhuyan et al. 2017). It is also difficult and costly for small organizations to implement data protection policies. In addition, the current focus of social media privacy and data security is self-governing. App users are adopting mobile technologies faster than providers can develop security (e.g. the HIPAA was approved in 1996 before mHealth development and continuous expansion). The General European Data Protection Regulation is recent, although regulations are still too general for mHealth applications (Martínez-Pérez et al. 2014). Martínez-Pérez et al. recommend actions to be taken on access control, authentication, security and confidentiality, integrity, informed consent, data transfer, data retention, BAN (Body Area Network) communication and breach notification.

Implication for practice 5.3
How do you keep the data on your computer secure? How aware are you regarding the ethical requirements in your workplace, and how well do you know the ethics approval process in your workplace?

Summary conclusion

Public health management and the health of the public have changed rapidly over the past century, and particularly over recent decades. Life expectancy has improved everywhere. Infectious diseases are no longer the leading causes of death worldwide. Chronic and non-communicable diseases, such as heart disease, cancers, diabetes, are now the global killers, and the poor suffer most. Using England as an example, public health and its structures struggle to find effective and sustainable ways to address non-communicable diseases and to have a more positive approach to health and health promotion. Partly, this is because of lack of resources in a difficult economic environment. Partly, it is because structures remain complex and fragmented. Digital technologies promise much, but structural digital developments have proved costly and delivery has been poor. Nevertheless, there are some promising developments, including in some low- and middle-income countries. There is a need for clear standards and good evaluation to bring sound ideas to maturity.

Digital technologies have also brought new kinds of public health problems, such as cyberbullying, data security, privacy and confidentiality issues. The growth of Big Data in a globalized connected world provides many opportunities, particularly in epidemiological research and practice. Big Data and crowdsourcing can help identify problems, patterns of health conditions, health needs assessment and priority areas for action. This can be empowering. Nevertheless, there are issues of choice and control in a neoliberal climate, as well as profound ethical issues which need to be addressed. The technology is running ahead of the policy analysis, and far ahead of strategies to improve practice. There is a need for co-ordinated efforts among all stakeholders in globalized communities. Training and education for the public health workforce are also important, so that practitioners can work efficiently in digitalized environments and are valued. Resources and support are also needed from policy makers to ensure quality and effective management of public health.

6

Digital Technology and Health Inequality

Key points

- To consider public policies in relation to health inequality in a digital environment.
- To understand nudge and choice architecture, as concepts and as policy tools in digital health promotion.
- To discuss health literacy, eHealth literacy and the digital divide.
- To discuss the digital access and digital ability of different groups of internet users.
- To discuss empowerment, and participation, in relation to health inequality and health equity in the context of digital health.

Introduction

Following on from the previous chapter on public health management, this chapter will focus on the implications of digital technology for health inequality. It will look critically at whether a widening health inequality gap might follow from the lack of accessibility and digital skills in the use of modern technologies among individuals and communities. Health inequality results from social inequality and is a longstanding societal issue. Evidence shows that the lower a person's social position, the worse their health is likely to be (Marmot 2010). The *European Health Report 2015* indicated that we are on track to achieve the Health 2020 target of reducing premature mortality – however, the health inequality gap remains wide, and much more can be done to reduce major risk factors (WHO 2015). Health and wellbeing are influenced by many social, economic and environmental determinants, as discussed in previous chapters. The WHO also states that health literacy is a critical determinant for health (WHO 2009, 2013, 2016). It announced its commitment to reduce health inequities for people of all ages, leaving no one behind in its Shanghai Declaration at the 2016 global health promotion conference (WHO 2016).

Reducing health inequalities is about fairness and social justice (WHO 2008; Marmot 2010). Income, wealth and power are linked to health inequalities. Laverack (2013) sees redistribution of power – transforming the unequal power relationship within and between societies – as key to addressing health inequalities. The WHO report (CSDH 2008) affirmed that poor social policies, unfair economic arrangements and bad politics are responsible for sustaining health inequalities. Addressing social, economic and environmental determinants is essential to achieving the United Nations Development Agenda 2030 and Sustainable Development Goals (WHO 2016). Facing a 'new global context for health promotion', unacceptable health inequities require global collective political action across many different sectors and regions.

Reducing health inequalities is a global agenda in which health service providers are turning to eHealth technologies for solutions to address barriers to health (WHO 2011a; Lewis 2012). Use of digital technologies in current health promotion is primarily based on individual responsibility, heavily linked to a market-driven western political agenda. As discussed in previous chapters, there are potentials and challenges in the use of digital technologies in health promotion for different population groups. For those with the abilities and resources, improved health and life chances might follow, compared with those without these advantages – e.g. lower-income groups, people living in rural communities, those with poor mental health, disabled people. New technologies might exacerbate inequality gaps. This chapter will critically discuss the use of digital technology in promoting health and reducing health inequality and health inequity. It will look at digital and health literacy and digital divides. Before we discuss digital technology and its effects on health inequality, we will look at public health policies in relation to health inequality, as well as nudge theory and choice architecture as a policy tool, before focusing our discussion on the impacts digital technology has on health inequality and how an ever-widening inequality gap can be reduced.

Healthy public policies and health inequality

The need to address health inequality and focus the promotion of health through addressing the social determinants of health has been highlighted throughout the world, e.g. the Marmot review in England (Marmot 2010); 'The social determinants of health 101 for healthcare: five plus five' in the USA (Magnan 2017); and the equity, social determinants and public health programmes of the WHO (WHO 2010). Healthy public policies and a health-supporting environment are needed for the promotion of good health. A co-ordinated integrated policy approach in service delivery involving all stakeholders and accommodating diverse needs is important (WHO 2011, 2016; Kwankam 2012; Marschang 2014). Health promotion is political (Dixey 2013; Cross et al. 2017). But there is a structural conflict between the values of health promotion (addressing health inequalities, promoting social justice, stressing mutuality and reciprocity) and the values of the marketplace (stressing individual consumption and competition). Health inequality is a global issue, and the top public health issues are similar in many countries, as seen in many WHO reports. This section focuses on how the UK deals with public health issues and addresses health inequality. Readers will need to reflect on their own country to understand how their government deals with health inequality and public health issues.

Although health promotion was widely discussed in the 1980s, prevention of ill health became more visible in government strategies in the 1990s. In the UK, the well-known Black Report on health inequality was published in 1980, but immediately discounted by the then incoming Conservative Thatcher government, a government strongly influenced by neoliberal thinking.

Individualism, the free market and privatization were all part of that government's policies (Baggott 2015). Many public health issues were raised during this period with the increased activities of pressure groups (O'Neil 2008). The important but contentious White Paper by the then Conservative government *The Health of the Nation* (Department of Health 1992) – a policy document that was target-orientated, based on a medical model of health, emphasizing a neoliberal ideology of individualism – set out its priority areas as coronary heart disease and strokes, cancer, accidents, mental illness, HIV/AIDS and sexual health. Cost-effectiveness was the major feature of managing health services. The following Labour government was determined to modernize the NHS. Its Public Health White Paper *Saving Lives: Our Healthier Nation* (Department of Health 1999) – the first time a government strategy acknowledged growing health inequality, accepting the Acheson Report (Acheson 1998) and social determinants of health as important to health improvement – focused on reducing death from cancer, coronary heart disease and stroke, accidents and mental illness, as well as smoking and obesity. However, it continued to be medically and target-orientated, and improvements were slow. In order to tackle public health issues, the 2004 *Choosing Health* White Paper (Department of Health 2004) again focused on similar priorities – smoking, obesity, physical activity, drinking, sexual health and mental health.

More recently, in 2010 – as in other developed countries – the UK's top three causes of premature death were heart disease, lung cancer and stroke. It was estimated that 70 per cent of total health and social care spending in England is for long-term conditions such as diabetes and heart diseases (Department of Health 2010a). The then Conservative-led Coalition government published another Public Health White Paper, *Healthy Lives, Healthy People* (HM Government 2010), building on the plans outlined in their *Equity and Excellence: Liberating the NHS Report* (Department of Health 2010b) and responding to the Marmot report *Fair Society, Healthy Lives* (Marmot 2010). It focused on improving health and wellbeing and tackling health inequalities, establishing the new Public Health England, providing leadership for public health services and ring-fencing public health budgets. It also included mental health, tobacco control, obesity and sexual health in the priorities.

The reorganization of public health functions in the UK meant that public health moved out of NHS management into local government. Informed by the Public Health Outcomes Framework, local health and wellbeing boards brought together local commissioners, local elective representatives, and Healthwatch and local consumer organizations to agree an integrated way to assess and meet local health needs and improve the health of the people in the locality, and to reduce premature mortality and inequality in health. This was a welcome move and most senior public health professionals agreed with this joint approach to commissioning public health services (Davies et al. 2016). However, according to the Commons Select Committee report on Public Health post-2013, the new system has proved more complex than anticipated – e.g. in roles and responsibilities, accountability and boundaries – causing fragmentation of service provision. There is potential conflict between political priorities within the local authority and clinical evidence-based decision making, e.g. in childhood obesity strategy and sexual health strategy. There is also fragmentation nationally, with public health responsibility divided between the Department of Health and NHS England, as well as other departments such as Health Education England and NICE (House of Commons Health Committee 2016).

Even though the government appears committed, in theory, to public health work and funding, disappointingly, it cut the public health budget by 7 per cent in 2015 (HM Government 2015; PHPSU 2015), followed by a 3.9 per cent per year cut over the following five years (HM Treasury 2015) – this at a time when health budgets were protected. In the latest public health policy documents, *NHS Five Year Forward View* (NHS 2014) and *Next Steps on the NHS Five Year Forward View* (NHS 2017), the Westminster government continues to stress its commitment on cancer care, mental illness, obesity, physical exercise, smoking and drinking. Only 5.29 per cent of the NHS budget in England was estimated for spending on prevention in 2014/15 (Davies et al. 2016). Financial pressures, as well as the loss of skilled public health workforce, are concerns. The evidence showing the cost-effectiveness of health promotion is strong, compared with the money spent on subsequent ill health in many areas. However, the restructuring of public health services in the UK has not produced any marked changes in outcomes. Davies et al. (2016) argue that where there is a change, it is difficult to tell whether it is because of system reform, budget cuts or societal factors. The continued cuts in public health budgets add to strain on service provision.

Currently, health inequality is being put on the list of 'burning injustices' by the present British Prime Minister Theresa May (House of Commons Health Committee 2016: 5). However, facing real-term cuts to public health budgets, practitioners are trying to deliver more with less. There is a growing mismatch between actual spending on public health and preventative action proposed in the *NHS Five Year Forward View* documents (Department of Health 2014, 2017). The select committee felt that this is a false economy and recognized that this would run the risk of widening the health inequality gap further (House of Commons Health Committee 2016).

It appears that, over the last twenty-five to thirty years, the same health issues have persisted globally, despite continuous government commitments and best efforts. The *NHS Five Year Forward View* (for England) made a strong commitment on a 'radical upgrade in prevention and public health' (NHS 2014: 3), admitting that the 'warning from the Wanless report in 2004 has not been heeded and the NHS is on the hook for the consequences'. According to *Next Steps on the NHS Five Year Forward View* (NHS 2017), more than one in three of us will get cancer in our lifetime. One in four of us will experience mental health problems. Tackling obesity, smoking and drinking is still a top priority globally. In addition, we are also facing challenges in tackling long-term conditions such as diabetes, dementia, mental health and supporting disabled people. With the problem of antimicrobial resistance, infectious diseases are still a risk, TB and multiple drug-resistant, sexually transmitted infections are also a threat (House of Commons Health Committee 2016). Health inequality and health inequity continue.

The concepts of nudge and choice architecture as policy tools in public health

Healthy public policy as an action area in the Ottawa Charter is important in health promotion. As already noted in previous chapters, government policies in the western world continue to be individual-focused, placing the responsibility of health on *individuals*, as shown in the use of new technology in promoting health, with very little emphasis on *structural* factors influencing health. Regulations, legislation, standards, partnership-working, self-regulations are all commonly used tools dependent on government ideologies, context and the socioeconomic environment, all depending on their related efficiency and effectiveness. One emphasis that has been used widely in the current neoliberal environment is the concept of 'nudge'. Based on the belief that people are not always rational and that their cognitive information-processing capacity is limited, 'nudge' as a policy concept originated from behaviour economics, asserted by Thaler and Sunstein (2008), moving people towards better decision making, giving rise to the role of a 'choice architect' who shapes environments in which people make decisions (Sugden 2009; Jung and Jeong 2011). The choice architects design ways to nudge people to make what the professionals see as healthy choices. In the UK, Thaler has been an advisor to the British government's Behavioural Insight team – the nudge unit – established by the Coalition government in 2010; and in the USA, Sunstein had worked for President Obama. Nudge is an approach, a government policy tool to steer people's behaviour towards making choices considered to be in their best interests – choices that they should make in an ideal situation. It should also be said that 'nudge' is not only being used in public health, it is widely used in commercial settings as a marketing technique to nudge people into making a particular choice.

Thaler and Sunstein (2008) discussed libertarian paternalism as a theoretical base for nudge. There is a balance between libertarianism – for preserving freedom of choice – and paternalism – for government intervention. Thaler and Sunstein see the co-existence of liberalism and paternalism as necessary, rather than contradictory. Paternalism can be seen as caring and considerate when people with more knowledge help those without. In a similar way, liberalism can also be seen as neglect – not taking responsibility for fellow citizens (Vallgarda 2012). Thaler and Sunstein (2008) argued that people have freedom to opt in or opt out as they choose. They claimed that their approach is about preserving liberty, and that their approach does not include regulations. It is only paternalistic in the sense of helping people to make better choices. However, Vallgarda (2012) argued that the nudge approach aligns well with paternalism and is not libertarian. It is a 'soft paternalism' that doesn't include coercion. Nudging people to make the 'correct' choice is not the same as leaving people to make their own free choices. For some, nudge can appear to interfere with personal lifestyle choices (Oliver 2013). Thaler claimed that nudges can be overt, and people are at liberty to ignore a nudge. However, Oliver argued that, if interventions are meant to influence unconscious action (the essence of nudge), how can one avoid the nudge? When a bottle of water is placed at eye level, not many of us would stop and think – wait a minute, I don't want to be nudged to pick up a healthy choice, so I will put the water back and pick up the bottle of Coke from the bottom shelf instead. An arguably earlier version of commercial 'nudge' (subliminal advertising) has been illegal in many countries for decades. The situation is similar in the digital environment, when there are so many health-related messages on the internet when you turn on the computer or when you look at your smartphone – e.g. food and drink advertisement (Boelsen-Robinson et al. 2015). For some, it is rather difficult to make the 'right' decision. This will be discussed further later, when we discuss eHealth literacy.

Wilkinson (2013) and Nys and Engelen (2017) discussed nudging and manipulation at length. Nys and Engelen agreed with Thaler and Sunstein (2008) that nudging is justified and legitimate. As in many public health strategies, whether something is ethical or not depends on your ethical point of view, as discussed in chapter 3. Goodwin (2012) saw nudge as deeply troubling, not empowering, unfair, manipulative, and to be rejected. He argued that people should be encouraged to think more collectively and to engage issues more deeply, to have the opportunity for citizen empowerment. One of the many criticisms of Thaler and Sunstein's libertarian paternalistic nudge was the lack of clear guidance on how better choices can be achieved. Their interpretation of liberalism and paternalism was also narrowly focused. The notion of nudge as a policy tool – where it nudges people towards a decision desired by the state, giving the impression that the expert knows best – is also being criticized (Sugden 2009; Jung and Jeong 2011). The complexity of the concept of 'choice' as discussed in chapter 3 also raises ethical concerns as to whether using choice architects and attempting to nudge people in their decision-making processes are acceptable. In addition, the focus of nudge on the individual and behavioural approach, ignoring structural factors, is also incompatible with the principles and practice of health promotion. The non-participatory way of decision making contradicts the empowerment concept in health promotion.

Reflection 6.1

Thinking about your own practice or your own interactions with friends and family – have you at any time nudged people to make choices you prefer? Do you think you are providing them with choices, or are you manipulating them to make a decision in line with your own choosing? How does this way of working compare with the empowerment approach to health promotion?

Health policies and health promotion

Health inequality is a global problem. In the USA, according to the national healthcare disparities report (Agency for Healthcare Research and Quality 2011), healthcare quality and access are suboptimal, especially for minority and low-income groups, also for women, older people, disabled people, and people living in rural areas. In the UK, according to the *Inequalities in Life Expectancy* report from The King's Fund (Buck and Maguire 2015), income-related inequalities have decreased. Although life expectancy has increased continuously in past decades, health inequality and health inequity continue to rise. Strategies for promoting health in the USA are similar to those in the UK. They are strongly behaviourally orientated. The main current focus is on individual action, choices and responsibility to improve health. Health behaviour modification strategies using health behaviour theories or social marketing strategies alone are inadequate for addressing health and social inequities, particularly for those in disadvantaged groups (Baum and Fisher 2014).

The success of health behaviour intervention by itself, without other means for health promotion, is unclear. Behaviour change can lead to stigmatizing and increase inequality, as it focuses on the person's behaviour rather than the cause of ill health. Any modest success has been for those at the top of the social gradient, and may even contribute to an increase in inequality (Laverack 2017). Baum and Fisher (2014) argued that universal strategies are not effective among people with lower socioeconomic status. Small-scale targeted strategies can produce some limited results, but are not cost-effective at large population level. The constraints of people's circumstances and their accumulated dispositions over their life course can be a barrier for behaviour change. The overall effect of behavioural strategy may even exacerbate health inequalities and be unsuccessful in improving health outcomes. As discussed in previous chapters, despite the acceptance of the social determinants of health, and the weak evidence on behaviour change strategies in reducing health inequality, government policies – such as those in the USA, Canada, the UK and Australia – still focus on the behavioural approach (Popay et al. 2010; Baum and Fisher 2014) and new technologies are mainly used for this purpose. Baum and Fisher (2014) argued that behavioural health promotion strategies are attractive to policy makers because of: the general strong focus and belief in recent years that see chronic illness as the result of poor lifestyle choices; the powerful driver of neoliberal ideology in western high-income free-market societies; those with the individualistic view of health possibly using power to protect their power relationship in these societies; the dominance of the medical model of health; and commercial industries and large corporations being able to sell 'solutions' to consumers. There is also a lack of leadership which makes inter-sectoral working difficult. Sustained community development strategies in disadvantaged areas are important in tackling social determinants and building local capacities for wellbeing (Baum and Fisher 2014).

In the UK, there is some evidence of leadership on policy in food advertising to children (WHO 2014); however, the third sector and academic communities still felt that the UK lacks adequate measures to protect children from the marketing of unhealthy food. Health campaigners believed online advertisers routinely breached general rules on food marketing. The continued preference for self-regulation has hindered the evolution of High Fat Sugar and/or Salt (HFSS) marketing restrictions. Ronit and Jensen (2014) found that self-regulatory codes were ineffective – they tend to be vague, and only resulted in small demonstrable effects. Boelsen-Robinson et al. (2015) agreed that the use of self-regulatory codes for food and drink marketing in the context of new media is limited. Tighter, mandatory regulations and commitment from the government are necessary (The Food Foundation 2017). Surveillance, monitoring and evaluation are critical to support effective action. Dedicated funding, effective leadership and a population- or community-based prevention strategy that includes multiple settings, multiple stakeholders and all levels of government are important (WHO 2012).

Health inequalities are socially and politically created. In the UK, the progress to reduce health inequalities is slow. Earlier policies solely targeting disadvantaged groups were not effective (Marmot 2010; Mackenzie et al. 2017). Earlier programmes such as Sure Start also ended before having a chance to demonstrate impact. There are, as well, other forces working against progress – e.g. the global economic system; fragmentation of health services; the erosion of the universalism of the social welfare system; regional and global labour market policies that affect employment (Whitehead and Popay 2010). Policies which identify where the problems lie and who is responsible for tackling them are better at addressing the issues. There is a disconnection between policy and the discussion of health inequality theory. Professionals also struggle to see inequalities in a wider societal context or think about innovative approaches (Mackenzie et al. 2017). Scott-Samuel and Smith (2015) agreed that a neoliberal approach prioritizing economic growth is a 'fantasy paradigm' that cannot realistically tackle health inequality. Even though there is a theoretical acknowledgement of the structural causes of health inequality, policies continue to be downstream, individualistic, outcome-focused and from a 'victim-blaming' behaviour change approach. It is increasingly so under the Conservative government (Mackenzie et al. 2017). Downstream preventative interventions tend to worsen the health inequality gap, unlike upstream interventions such as provision of resources and fiscal interventions (Lorenc et al. 2012).

Digital technology used in health strongly aligns with a neoliberal approach to managing health. As we have shown, it encourages people to become responsible citizens, taking responsibility for their own health, e.g. via mobile technologies, wearable technologies, health apps. Any evidence for digital interventions reducing health inequalities and inequities is lacking. Currently, the UK government continues to reaffirm its promotion of healthy communities, with no evidence of impact, making use of digital technology and new models of care to detect and treat people with high-risk conditions. Indeed, *Next Steps on the NHS Five Year Forward View* (NHS 2017) has a whole chapter on integrated local services such as STP (Sustainability and Transformation Partnership), accountable care services, and Multispecialty Community Providers. It discussed partnership between GPs, community health, hospital services, rehabilitation services and local government departments, such as housing, leisure and transport. Fundamentally, there is no real discussion of or guidance on how exactly it would address the factors affecting health. Disappointingly, it is still a policy paper focusing on a medicalized and downstream approach to health, based on individualistic behaviour approaches and lifestyle interventions, rather than addressing the social determinants of health based on the social model of health, addressing the causes of ill health and health inequality.

Reflection 6.2

If you have experience as a health promotion professional, have you had a role in the policy-making process? Do you have the power to influence policy? Can you give three examples of how you influence policy decisions?

Digital health and health inequality

The changing landscape of Web 2.0 interventions is challenging traditional health promotion. It provides huge opportunities for health providers in the design of healthcare strategies and interventions. However, inequality of access is a key issue for, among others, people with low income and lacking resources, ethnic minorities, older people, people with mental health needs, disabled people, people who live in rural areas, people with low digital and literacy skills, and so-called 'hard to reach' groups (Marschang 2014). Internet access is strongly correlated to age, education and income level, and geographic location. There are also those who do not want to be 'empowered consumers' of healthcare. Some people may not want to have the intrusion of technology in their everyday lives. Existing social inequities and poor health can be exacerbated by lack of knowledge or access to digital technology (Lupton 2012, 2013a, 2015c).

With more widely available electronic and mobile devices and faster broadband, competitively priced, the accessibility gap, although significant, is starting to narrow. However, many people still don't have access to the internet. The *Exploring the Digital Nation* report by the National Telecommunications and Information Administration in the USA (US Department of Commerce 2013) showed a stubborn presence of digital divide by socioeconomic status, race/ethnicity and urbanity. Engagement of eHealth with the public is also a concern (Chou et al. 2013). Silva et al. (2018) found that people in more educated, wealthy and older households living in urban areas with more broadband providers are more likely to have fixed broadband subscriptions. The high number of older households using fixed broadband through traditional technologies could be because younger people are more likely to use mobile broadband. The lack of broadband availability can be a hindrance. They also found that broadband adoption rates among African-American households in their study are lower in both urban and rural areas.

Medically underserved populations, such as those living in poverty, are often seen as having limited *access* to health information. People with a medical condition that limits travel, rural residents and Black and Minority Ethnic (BME) groups were less likely to access and use the internet. They also mainly accessed the internet from home (Wang et al. 2011). A study by Zach et al. in the USA (2011) found that the lack of internet access itself is not a primary barrier to health information. Mobile phone technology could provide accessible communication with groups, and provide targeted health promotion services. But the digital divide is at the level of information *use* rather than information *access*. It's about skills in using the internet and wider aspirational and life skills. A study by Chen (2013) on the relationship between internet access and social capital found that younger, white, better-educated, more affluent, employed, urban and suburban Americans remain more likely to access and use the internet than older, black, less-educated, less-affluent, unemployed and rural Americans. According to Chen (2013), there is a link between social connectivity and digital connectivity. Bonding people with resources (people who know how to use the internet) could narrow digital divides. Bonding social capital with strong ties in a homogeneous group is positively associated with online communication, helping to reduce digital divides (Chen 2013). The study also shows that most social interaction remains local, within people's intimate bonding network, even though technology has enhanced communication at great geographical and social distance. Bridging social capital is useful for internet access, whereas resource-rich bonding capital is useful for promoting internet use and online communication. However, bonding social capital is unevenly distributed and takes time to develop. Thus, community initiatives would be useful in promoting the skills of disadvantaged groups in the use of mobile phones, through informal mentoring and training.

Looking at the usage of digital technology, it is relatively easy for organizations to provide health services using voice or text communication through conventional networks, but much harder to use internet for health surveillance, public health awareness, and services that support decision making, as these services require enhanced capabilities and infrastructure lacking in many organizations, e.g. the NHS in the UK. We also need to take into consideration life aspiration, literacy skills, connectivity and accessibility issues such as bandwidth, affordability, people's impairments and technophobia (WHO 2011a). From a sociological perspective, despite the claim that wearable technologies are inert, neutral objects used to collect health data in the interest of healthcare, these devices are seen as actively shaping the lives of the people who use them. Digital technologies are not politically neutral, but rather are implicated in a dense web of power relationships (Lupton 2015c).

Health inequality in the context of eHealth is an area that has not been fully examined (Marschang 2014). A central part is played by eHealth in facilitating socioeconomic inclusion and patient empowerment through greater transparency, and access to information and services (European Commission 2012). However, the fast-changing landscape of eHealth, the costs involved, the digital literacy skills needed and the plethora of information on the web present challenges and barriers for many. The lack of co-ordination, financial resources, and uneven infrastructure and interoperability also present many challenges for enthusiastic professionals. Although the accessibility gap in digital technology is narrowing slowly, the knowledge gap between proficient and inept users is getting wider. The social inequality gap is widened by who can *make use* of the internet, not just who can *access* it (Marschang 2014). This is a fundamental divide. There is also a need to understand how social media can affect attitudes, beliefs and health outcomes, and a need to design methods for evaluation and measurement of success. The disparities between different target populations also need to be assessed, and the participatory nature of social media needs to be harnessed – e.g. observational research to evaluate the role of user-generated content and information accuracy can be useful (Chou et al. 2013). Data security is also important and well-designed integrated healthcare management systems, with collaboration among service providers, and supporting strategies, policies and adequate resources, are needed (WHO 2011a).

Implication for practice 6.1

Think about the use of digital technology and its impact on health inequality – how could you ensure your clients have equal opportunity to access the internet and have the skills to participate in your digital interventions?

Health literacy and the digital divide

Health literacy is a critical determinant of health (WHO 2013, 2016; IUHPE 2018; Trezona et al. 2018; Sykes and Wills 2018) and an emergent public health issue. Until recently, most evidence on health literacy has come from the USA, mainly on functional health literacy (a patient's ability to understand prescriptions, appointments, medicine labels, and manage chronic conditions). This narrow interpretation of basic functional health literacy has been a barrier for educating patients about their chronic illness, and represents a major cost to healthcare (Nutbeam 2000; Van den Broucke 2014). It is being seen as insufficient in promoting health behaviour and for health promotion. Health literacy involves more than just reading and understanding information. It involves finding, understanding, evaluating and communicating information for informed decision making (Nutbeam 2000; WHO 2009; Coleman et al. 2011; Pleasant et al. 2011; Mackert et al. 2016). Berkman et al. (2010: 16) defined health literacy as 'The degree to which individuals can obtain, process, understand, and communicate about health-related information needed to make informed health decisions.' They recognized that language, culture and social capital, as well as health information technology, have a role to play in how we define health literacy.

The 7th Health Promotion Conference in Nairobi identified the importance of health literacy. The focuses at the conference were on access to information through ICT; increased use of health information through empowerment; increasing the flow of information through multi-sectoral collaboration; and developing appropriate ways to measure and report progress in improving health literacy levels (WHO 2009). Health literacy is also one of the three action areas in the Shanghai Charter on Health Promotion (WHO 2016). According to the WHO, there are three distinct levels of health literacy:

- functional level, as in reading and writing;
- conceptual literacy, with skills and competencies to seek out, comprehend, evaluate and use health information, to make informed choices, reducing health risk and increasing quality of life; and
- health literacy as empowerment, where active citizenship is strengthened for health, involving individuals in understanding their rights as patients and their ability to navigate through the healthcare system, acting as informed consumers regarding health risks and options in healthcare, and able to improve health through political means.

Nutbeam (2000) similarly classifies health literacy into three levels:

- basic functional literacy, as described by WHO (2009);
- communicative/interactive literacy, such as cognitive and social skills whereby one can participate in everyday activities such as extracting information, deriving meaning and applying this to changing circumstances; and
- critical literacy, where one can critically analyse information, helping in gaining greater control over life events. It encompasses both action and agency, applying information critically, but also individual and community political action on social determinants of health in pursuit of social justice (Sykes and Wills 2018). However, Sykes and Wills's evaluation shows that the political action element of critical health literacy is the least well understood by their participants.

From a medical point of view, health literacy is seen as a *risk factor*: low health literacy is associated with poor health outcomes. Medical professionals struggle with their own lack of competence here. For them, low-literacy patients are a problem (Nutbeam 2008; Coleman et al. 2016). However, high-literacy patients are seen as a different problem. From a public health and health promotion point of view, good health literacy is framed positively as an *asset*, a social capital to be strengthened (Nutbeam 2008; WHO 2013). It helps build resilience among individuals and communities, and shapes the sociocultural context in which people live. Linking to the discussion on power and empowerment in chapter 3, health literacy is rooted in the health promotion movement, aiming to empower people, and is an essential dimension of strengthening health systems. Navigating complex healthcare systems can be challenging, and health information is often poorly presented. Recorded phone messages are usually rapidly spoken. The operator can't answer questions. There is usually a long wait for the phone to be answered. People can't find their way round healthcare facilities. Health professionals often speak in medical jargon. Directions for use and warnings on prescriptions are often unclear. As regards digital health, web-based information is generally designed for aesthetic appearance rather than usefulness. Health promotion messages should be tailored and well designed in partnership with communities. Quality assurance systems should be established to prevent misinformation and miscommunication (WHO 2013).

With consumerism and free-market economies in modern society, it can be difficult for people, even those well educated, to navigate through health information to improve their health, even though literacy and health literacy are fundamental for healthy living. Around half of US adults have low health literacy (Mackert et al. 2016). Half of the adults in eight European countries also have inadequate health literacy skills (European Health Literacy Consortium 2012). Vulnerable groups, such as older people, ethnic minorities, recent immigrants, and those with low levels of education and low income are worse off, with limited health literacy. Improving health literacy needs a whole-society approach involving multiple stakeholders. A study on networks and interest groups in health literacy, Sorensen et al. (2018), suggests that there is a vibrant worldwide health literacy community driving the rise of an emerging global health literacy movement for social change towards empowerment and health equity. The European health policy framework aims to promote empowerment and participation of people in their communities and in their healthcare. Its conceptual model of health literacy covers individuals' or the community's abilities in accessing, understanding, appraising and applying information (Sorensen et al. 2012).

Measuring health literacy is also difficult. Health literacy, both individual and collective, needs to be measured and monitored (WHO 2013). Measuring health literacy is a dynamic process and there are few satisfactory measuring tools (Berkman et al. 2010). There are several health literacy scales. The commonly used ones, such as the Rapid Estimate of Adult Literacy in Medicine (REALM) and the Test of Functional Health Literacy in Adults (TOFHLA), are both inadequate. The Health Activity Literacy Scale (HALS) shows some promise, but has limitations as it excludes oral skills, lacks problem-solving tests and does not measure attitudes, values and beliefs (WHO 2009). Measurement should also be a regular process. Existing measures are too individualized and need collective-level measures, as well as to rate the literacy-friendliness of material, organizations and environments (WHO 2013). Pleasant et al. (2011) proposed that measures of health literacy need to be based on sound theory, able to measure the health literacy of individuals as well as of health systems and health professionals (both information-seekers and the information-givers). It should also include comparison across context, culture, life course, population group and research setting. Calling for global action to improve health literacy in the population, the IUHPE global working group on health literacy identifies four priorities and action areas in health literacy, relating to: health promotion policy, appropriate intervention, measurement and research, and building capacity with an intersectorial approach (IUHPE 2018).

eHealth literacy

The rapid adoption of digital technology provides great opportunities but the uncontrollable, non-moderated and viral nature of the social web poses high risks of misinformation and disinformation. The volume of rapidly produced content also has implications for health and digital literacy skills. People need to learn to access, critically assess and appraise information on the web (WHO 2013). Mackert et al. (2016) found that people with low health literacy were less likely to use health information technology tools or perceive them as easy or useful. They associated the use of conventional health technology with greater perceptions of privacy. They also had a lower trust of government media and technology companies, but put more trust in health providers. Hence, there is a need for governments to work with health providers in the development of health information technologies. A participatory approach in building information pages is important to ensure no one is left behind (WHO 2013). Web use should be robust to ensure web quality, aligning with the values and principles of public good, for example following the guidance on the *Health on the Net (HON) Code of Conduct for Medical and Health Web Sites* (Health on the Net Foundation 2013).

Digital technologies are important in gaining access to many services in daily life, such as for information, employment, housing, education, social networking, banking, etc. Health services around the world are increasing the use of technology for communication in order to improve service provision. This can have potential impacts on existing health inequalities and inequities as both the private sector and government rely on technology-mediated services for support and information (Baum et al. 2012). As more advantaged groups continue to have good digital access, disadvantaged groups are being left behind. This digital exclusion is leading to a steeper social and health gradient. The ability of highly eHealth-literate people to extract benefit leads to a new inequality in digital health information. Improving health literacy is important in reducing health inequality, as well as reducing societal cost (WHO 2013). Equity in electronic health literacy needs to be enhanced and ensured. Health literacy empowers individuals and enables their engagement in health promotion action.

Information-seeking on the net is largely an independent goal-driven activity without guidance from health professionals. There is a plethora of health information on the internet. The quality of online health information can be variable (Chesser et al. 2015). Disparities in health information access persist particularly among those with insufficient skills to discriminate between credible and fraudulent online health information (Stellefson et al. 2017). To ensure health promotion intervention is effective, it is essential that methods to communicate health messages are appropriate. In order to use electronic methods to communicate messages effectively, people need to be able to work with technology, and have the ability to access, understand and process health information for meaningful decision making (Norman and Skinner 2006). A study by McElhinney et al. (2018) on the use of avatars – virtual representations of participants in a social virtual environment – showed that participants developed and used their social skills and cultural competencies to access and be able to appraise information in multiple formats in their virtual world. It showed an impact on their literacy practice and helped to influence their behaviour change in their physical world. McElhinney et al. found that there was an improvement of individual and community literacy practice. They also found that the interaction participants can have as an avatar with their peers and professionals in the virtual world was useful. There was a learning of sharing, relationship-building, networking and negotiating skills. They also reported changes of attitude, reduced stress and anxiety, improved social skills, increased empathy and a positive influence on the self-management of their long-term conditions, such as lifestyle changes. The virtual world acted as a place for people with limiting functional or psychosocial capacity to rehearse their learning before attempting it in the physical world, as discussed in chapter 2. However, the design and navigation issues of the virtual environment need to be considered and tested carefully.

Using Bourdieu's concept of capital and field – competition and interactions between different social, economic and cultural capitals shaping the distribution of power in a society – Baum et al. (2012) conceptualize the digital world as a societal field where there is struggle for resources and where power is unevenly distributed. They found that people who are already disadvantaged in their access to economic, social and cultural capital are further excluded and lack power in the digital field, as they have insufficient capital to accrue more. Hence, people with inadequate educational opportunities are disempowered and feel further excluded in the digital field. It's a vicious circle in which lack of knowledge in using digital technology further lowers the ability to gain access to resources. As seen in the discussion of power and empowerment in chapter 3, low educational opportunities lead to low fundamental literacy, which also shapes health literacy and in turn affects people's ability to improve their health, thus disempowering them. Breaking the cycle of deprivation requires effort in lifting people out of their poverty trap. Maintaining equity in health promotion practice requires breaking the digital literacy cycle, so that access is more inclusive; provision of opportunities is needed to improve people's capital (Baum et al. 2012), e.g. reducing the cost of software and hardware, providing free WiFi, improving education, employment, digital skills training for everyone. There is a need for health promoters to understand the barriers posed by the interaction of digital literacy with health and fundamental literacy. Support should be provided based on people's needs, to ensure digital inclusion and maintain health equity (Baum et al. 2012) – e.g. non-digital forms of communication may need to continue. Baum et al. (2012) argued that health services going paperless may not always be appropriate.

Norman and Skinner (2006) defined eHealth literacy as the ability to seek, find, understand and appraise health information from electronic sources and apply the knowledge gained to addressing or solving health problems. People with greater eHealth literacy are more able to make informed health decisions. Six core skills make up eHealth literacy – traditional, health, information, scientific, media and computer literacies (Norman and Skinner 2006; WHO 2013). There are very few eHealth literacy scales measuring electronic health literacy. A commonly used one would be the eHEALS (eHealth Literacy Scale), a patient-reported tool, originally developed by Norman and Skinner (2006) as an assessment tool to measure the level of eHealth literacy skill. Despite wide use in different countries globally, there are some challenges. A study by Richtering et al. (2017) on health literacy and eHealth literacy in patients with cardiovascular disease showed that eHEALS is generally sufficient, with some limitations – e.g. regarding using eHealth and understanding eHealth. A telephone interview conducted by Stellefson et al. (2017) with older adults on their eHealth literacy also found that the eHEALS, with some modifications, produced sufficient reliable measures reflecting societal shifts in online health information-seeking among older people. Similarly, Paige et al.'s (2017) study on eHealth literacy and people with chronic ill health also found that the eHEALS is reliable in measuring the self-reported eHealth literacy among this group of people. Healthcare providers can use eHEALS scores to identify patients who need training to enhance their eHealth literacy.

Implication for practice 6.2
When designing health promotion interventions, how might you assess the literacy level (including eHealth literacy) of your clients? What are your roles (in terms of health inequality and inequity) in ensuring that health messages can reach, and be understood and used by, your clients?

Different groups of internet users

According to the Office for National Statistics (2014) and Ofcom (2014, 2015), access to the internet among people who have less confidence in using digital technology is increasing rapidly. However, 12 per cent of the population are unable to access the internet and have no plans to do so in the near future (the self-excluded group) (Coulter and Mearns 2016). People who are digitally excluded tend to be those with greater health needs, such as older people, disabled people, people with chronic health conditions, etc. (Honeyman et al. 2016). A systematic review by Chesser et al. (2015) looked at eHealth literacy among under-served populations who may have decreased access to health infrastructure and technology in the USA. It was found that most studies did not assess the impact of locality on eHealth literacy, and those that did assess it were predominantly in urban areas. There is a gap in the literature regarding underserved popula-tions and eHealth literacy, particularly those in rural areas. While digital technology is becoming more common worldwide, with two-thirds of UK citizens using smartphones to access the internet (Ofcom 2015) and more people acquiring skills in using online health services (Coulter and Mearns 2016), nevertheless almost a quarter of UK adults (23 per cent) lack basic digital skills, and 11 per cent have never used the internet (Good Things Foundation 2016).

The digital divide exists between different demographic groups. The improvement of health information technology (HIT) is useful if service users can engage with these systems (Ennis et al. 2012). The internet could be particularly useful for housebound people and older adults with chronic conditions, for the management of their health issues, for daily activities such as shopping and banking, as well as for social networking, keeping in touch with family and friends. It is estimated that a third to half of the people in developed countries have difficulties in understanding and engaging in healthcare (Raynor 2012). People with chronic conditions often lack skills to navigate and identify relevant health information online. They also tend to be older (Paige et al. 2017). Some people may have a carer who has high health literacy and eHealth literacy to help them with daily activities, but many don't. Older people with chronic ill health, with a high degree of functional impairment and limited financial resources, who are housebound, have a lower education level, and those with cognitive decline, computer and technology phobia, poor internet network access, and generally lacking self-efficacy, are an importantly excluded group. Despite the increasing availability of eHealth resources, it is still difficult for some people to find, understand and benefit from health information services (Milne et al. 2014).

A study by Choi and DiNitto (2013), comparing groups of older adults and younger groups, both low-income and homebound, found both groups to be low internet users (only 34 per cent of the younger and 17 per cent of the older group). The main reasons are cost or their disabilities. Also, within this low-income group of housebound people, racial/ethnic minorities and those with lower income are much less likely to use the internet – however, they did express interest in using it. Activity of Daily Living and Instrumental Activity of Daily Living impairments are barriers to internet use. These low-income and homebound internet users, whether older or younger, have a pattern of internet usage similar to the general population. Younger people use the internet for a wider variety of activities, whereas older people's usages were much narrower. As expected, older people had less confidence and lower self-efficacy in internet use; participants who lived alone and had higher incomes had higher efficacy levels. The authors also found lower levels of eHealth efficacy in both groups, and less willingness to join online discussion groups. This could be due to confidentiality concerns. Financial support or allowances provided to acquire computers, as well as education, can help increase use of the internet among disadvantaged groups. Better computer and software design can also help people with severe disabilities.

Exposure and practice increase computer-use skills, and people with low efficacy can be helped to learn how to use the internet.

As discussed, eHealth Literacy levels tend to be higher among younger and better-educated people. In a study using eHEALS on eHealth literacy of primary lung cancer survivors, who are usually older, less educated, with poorer health, Milne et al. (2014) found that lung cancer survivors' eHealth literacy is generally low. Few survivors think the internet is useful for health decision making, yet they felt it's important to access health information on the net. People who can access eResources easily and have higher educational attainment have a higher eHealth literacy score, whereas people with lower eHealth literacy get less benefit from eResources, even though they had access. Interestingly, they found no significant association here between eHealth literacy and age. There was also no significant association between self-perceived health status and eHealth literacy. However, they found that people with chronic illnesses did have lower eHealth literacy levels. Improving health literacy is important for lung cancer survivors as many can survive longer with better treatment, but also have other health complications and need access to health decision-making resources.

Digital technology can also be very useful in the area of mental health, as discussed in chapter 2. A study by Ennis et al. (2012) found that technological access and use among mental health internet users are similar to those of the general population. It appears that physical rather than mental conditions are more of a barrier in accessing technology. Older people had lower knowledge, access and use, as well as lower confidence about modern technologies such as smartphones. Women also have less confidence in mobile phone use. They also found that BME groups access computers remotely (rather than at home) more than white participants. Ennis et al. suggest that computer-based technology is the most appropriate format to facilitate engagement with mental health users. Resources and skills with extra support should be provided particularly for the older group and the BME group.

Implication for practice 6.3
Thinking about the principles and value of health promotion – e.g. participation and empowerment – what is your role in ensuring your clients have equal opportunities in accessing, understanding and using healthcare resources?

Empowerment, participation, health inequality and health equity

Helping people to improve their eHealth literacy skills encourages people to participate and take control of their own health. This is important in narrowing the digital divide and promoting empowerment. In order to reduce inequality and health inequity, interventions need to meet the needs of the people. Empowerment and participatory approaches to health promotion appear throughout this book. This is a fundamental principle in health promotion, as discussed in depth in chapter 3. The interactiveness of Web 2.0 technology, promoting two-way communication, provides opportunities for people to contribute in health matters, participating in the decision making in their own health career and promoting empowerment, as well as for professionals working together with the public (Hanson et al. 2008). As shown by Green et al.'s empowerment/participation gradient (2015), empowerment and participation are positively associated with each other; higher levels of participation lead to higher levels of empowerment.

A study by Sarkar et al. (2011), investigating the use of an internet-based patient portal for diabetic patient self-management, found that older, less-educated and some BME groups were less likely to request a password and to go onto the portal. Similarly, in a small study by Thompson and Kumar (2011) in an urban clinic, the authors found that, although a high proportion of their clients used the internet, only a third accessed the internet sufficiently to make it important for patient education. They did find text messaging was more commonly used among African Americans, females and younger patients in their practice area in managing clinic appointments. Despite increased access and use of health information via the internet, one must be cautious when designing internet-based interventions and not overestimate internet use for clinical purposes. A collaborative approach with policy makers, health practitioners, web developers and, most importantly, people themselves in designing health promotion interventions is needed to ensure interventions are fit for their purposes.

The internet as an information-provision tool is very useful for health promotion in enabling and empowering informed decision making. It can provide support and shared personal experience with other web users, helping people gain confidence and improve their self-efficacy in managing their own health. However, poorly developed websites may lead to misinformation or misuse of information. A study of electronic food vouchers from the World Food Programme showed that technology has the potentially negative consequences of excluding some individuals from access to assistance – e.g. illiterate or older persons – while also creating positive effects in the increased security of cash and vouchers. Technology has the potential to deliver cash quickly and safely, but in countries without good infrastructure and organization, technology can create more problems for beneficiaries, for example in locations where internet outages delayed cash collection (Berg et al. 2013). Kelly et al. (2015) developed a tool to help website developers, health professionals and researchers with website development, the presentation of information and the kinds of materials that are useful for web users.

Service users need to be involved in managing and commissioning their own healthcare, a participatory approach encouraging citizen participation in healthcare. For example, service users can have direct control over their own care package, managing it through the local authority, through a third-party support organization or by themselves. However, in the digital world, not all patients have the material resources or technical competence to take responsibility for their care. Democratization of healthcare can leave people further disempowered, marginalized and isolated (Horrocks and Johnson 2014). Similarly to Horrocks and Johnson, Frohlich and Abel (2013) argued that social inequalities are socially structured and unfair. Epidemiological approaches to health behaviour, targeted at individuals but ignoring their social context, are a problem as behaviour is socially orientated. Some people live in environments where they may have unequal and limited choice. Studies of inequality need to move from studying the inequality of health outcomes to studying the inequity of opportunities that leads to health inequalities, as discussed in chapter 4 (Frohlich and Abel 2013).

According to Salutogenic theory (Antonovsky 1979, 1987) – the sense of coherence (SOC) model of health concept as discussed in chapter 3 – health is a relative concept: people learn to cope with stressful situations and stay well. People having generalized resistance resources (GRRs), such as money, knowledge, experience, social support, etc., are more able to cope with stressors. People with high SOC have stronger abilities to manage stress and are more satisfied with their lives and enjoy a higher level of quality of life (Lindstrom and Eriksson 2010). Antonovsky saw it as the responsibility of society to create conditions that foster the strength of coping, the SOC. A good society is one where people care about each other, not simply about having personal choices. Empowerment and participation are central elements of Salutogenesis and can be seen as tools to enhance individual SOC (Lindstrom and Eriksson 2010). Lindstrom and Eriksson see that the Salutogenic approach, together with the concept of resilience against stress and ill health as discussed by Rutter (1980), could be a guide for public health, e.g. in social and mental wellbeing, by focusing on the prerequisites for quality of life and promoting good health. It would be much more important to develop societies and life conditions focusing on the creation of settings where we all have the opportunity to live well.

Web 2.0 technologies give rise to people as prosumers who produce and consume digital content at the same time in their participatory experience of the interactive web platform, e.g. social media sites provide a platform for people to share their experience and knowledge with others, supporting each other in self-care or self-management of their health, developing collaborative relationships with professionals as well as providing data as part of the Big Data phenomenon, for example via crowdsourcing, data harvesting, data assemblage, as discussed in the previous chapters (Ritzer et al. 2012; Lupton 2014a). On one hand, this can promote empowerment and participatory approaches to healthcare. People are encouraged to participate and take control of their own health destiny. They become expert patients, contributing by supporting each other. However, the commercial and research value of these user-generated data means that activities, e.g. crowdsourcing, can also be exploited by web developers which Lupton called 'the digital patient experience economy'. The commodification and commercialization of these activities rarely involve users in designing or developing their website platform or applications, nor do users have any control over the final product (Lupton 2014a). Co-production of health requires an equal partnership and an equal power relationship where people work together with professionals, with the goal of creating health on a level playing field, in a health-supporting environment. The values for co-production, as described by the Coalition for Collaborative Care, include ownership and understanding of co-production by all, a culture of openness and honesty, a commitment to sharing power and decisions with citizens, clear communication, and a culture in which people are valued and respected (C4CC 2014). Only with real participation (throughout the whole decision-making process, from proposal development and service design to the evaluation and reporting journey) can this be empowering.

Reflection 6.3

If you have experience as a health promotion professional – how do you involve your clients? What level of involvement do you employ? Do you think digital technology improves your service provision? How do you involve your clients if new technology is to be used as part of your services? How do you ensure health equity in your practice?

Summary conclusion

As mentioned in the introduction, income, wealth and power are linked to health inequalities. Poorer groups do not have an equal share in improvements in lifestyle, as compared with wealthier groups. The current UK government may seek an integrated approach, as seen with the emphasis on prevention in the *NHS Five Year Forward View* paper (NHS 2014), but it is also important to take into account local knowledge, history and experience if the improvement is to continue (Buck and Maguire 2015). Buck and Maguire from The King's Fund argued for a more coherent health programme and wider policy approach from government.

Web 2.0 technology provides huge opportunities and possibilities for health promotion. It is not only a 'digitized library', but rather a 'vibrant social universe' where people communicate with each other as online communities (Gibbons et al. 2011). Gibbons et al. suggest an ecological approach, addressing individual, provider and system issues to ensure the full potential of digital technology. For individuals, the challenges remain of health literacy, language, integration of evidence-based information, resources and access to complex interventions. Emerging evidence suggests minority populations may be more responsive to social media.

Uptake of mobile technology, developing digital health that can be delivered via mobile devices, could be useful. For service providers, technology can help provide enhanced support for clinical decisions at the point of care and research, improve clinical care and health research, as well as facilitate greater user participation in the care process, meeting the needs of the population to reduce health inequality and promoting health equity.

Health inequality is reducible, avoidable and multifaceted. As discussed in the report of the eHealth Stakeholder Group (Marschang 2014), Marschang agreed with Gibbons et al. (2011) that problems can be experienced at individual, professional and health-system levels. At the individual level, the problems lie with the accessibility and affordability of technology, its usability and appropriateness, as well as people's own digital health literacy. For professionals, eHealth technologies do not exist in isolation. They compete for resources in a changing health system and a wider environment of 'austerity'. This is also a time in which demography and disease are reshaping what is meant by health, care and treatment. In all of this, the roles of health and care professionals are challenging and changing. For us to benefit from the potentials of eHealth technology successfully in practice, continuous investment, nurturing and training will be required. The eHealth Stakeholder Group suggested the following were needed (Marschang, 2014: 4):

- Improve access to eHealth and involve all stakeholders
- Accommodate diverse needs and reduce technological pressure
- Improve digital health literacy
- Integrate eHealth into overall health and social care system policy
- Evaluate the impact of eHealth solutions and build up an evidence base
- Give specific consideration to empowering patients with disabilities / specific diseases
- Consider financial subsidies for the purchase of eHealth equipment / ICT access.

7

Looking to the Future

Introduction

This chapter will draw a summary conclusion to the book. It will discuss the future potentials and challenges that a digital society will face as we go into the era of Web 3.0 digital and the Internet of Things. With the fast pace of development of digital technology, we need to look at the world afresh. Although the Digital Age should not be assumed to be the Promised Land, there are many possibilities for promoting population health, reducing health inequalities via individual and community empowerment, as well as ensuring an efficient and effective public health service. There are also challenges to be considered, such as data sharing and data security; addressing the social, economic, ethical and political implications; the underlying cause of social and health inequalities; the structural barriers for health; promoting health in low- and middle-income countries of the Global South (Piette et al. 2012); as well as addressing the power relationship imbalance, including whose voices are heard and whose are ignored (WHO 2011a; Lupton 2015a), as discussed in this book.

The future of internet interventions lies in their dissemination potential (Bennett and Glasgow 2009). For eHealth to be sustainable, a well-planned, co-ordinated and integrated approach is needed. In order to learn for the future, evaluation of eHealth programmes is essential (WHO 2011a). A health-focused, participatory research agenda is needed if the implementation of eHealth programmes is to be successful for the development of evidence-based practice, and for the promotion of equity and social justice in health (Van Heerden et al. 2012). Training and education are also needed to ensure the use of digital technology reaches its highest potential. This chapter will end with some recommendations for practitioners, commissioners and all relevant stakeholders on the successful use of digital technologies in promoting the health of the public.

Further development of digital technology for health

The provision of health service is a complex business, in the UK or elsewhere. The use of digital technology can no doubt improve health for many individuals and communities, enhancing health services provision through empowerment, research and better decision-making processes. Technological advances can promote health and health-related activities, as discussed in chapter 2. There are many opportunities and possibilities. It is hoped that new technologies can transform healthcare, leading to cost-effective and improved quality of care, and positive health outcomes (National Information Board 2014). However, a systematic review by Black et al. (2011) showed that there is a lack of evidence to show eHealth is cost-effective or improves health outcomes. Grady et al. (2018) agreed that harnessing eHealth and mHealth technologies to improve public health has been challenging, and evidence supporting the effectiveness of technology-based interventions in addressing non-communicable diseases remains varied. A lack of initial and sustained engagement of users is a key constraint (Birnbaum et al. 2015). The evidence base for popular apps and their information quality is also questionable (Grady et al. 2018). Coulter and Mearns (2016) suggested that immediate cost-effectiveness of eHealth is probably a naïve hope. Careful design may deliver efficiency only in the longer term. The potential for eHealth in improving health systems and safety, quality and efficiency was acknowledged in a World Health Assembly resolution in 2005 (WHO 2005a). It is therefore important that interventions should be designed properly and evaluated comprehensively to provide evidence for practice.

British healthcare systems are slow in embracing technology as compared with other sectors of the UK economy. The UK governments are committed, but healthcare systems are complex. Digitizing health services needs time and resources across the country, so that service provision is co-ordinated and aligned with the wider systems. Time scales need to be realistic, both for the technology to embed into the existing complex system and for adoption by people within the system. Overambitious goals can be a hindrance. It is also unclear where resources, investment and support will come from (Coulter and Mearns 2016; Honeyman et al. 2016). In an age of austerity, the lack of clarity in investment from government can be a barrier. There is a need for more sustainable sources of funding, greater support for the adoption of new technologies, and better ways to evaluate impact (Lewis et al. 2012).

The concern over security of online personal data, and the reluctance of professionals to hand over control, have not helped progress (National Information Board 2014; Mudge et al. 2015). A qualitative metasynthesis by Mudge et al. (2015) on clinicians' view of their role in self-management of long-term conditions found that clinicians appeared to wrestle with the issues of control, moving from a hierarchical dominant medical model of practice to person-centred care. There is a tension between ensuring patients' best interests versus patient choices and responsibility. Participation and collaborative practice are fundamental to health promotion, and the foundation for empowering approaches to health. Partnership is needed among health professionals, technology developers and the people using the system for successful implementation, particularly in ensuring technologies are fit for purpose (Coulter and Mearns 2016).

In their review, Coulter and Mearns (2016) suggest three principles for achieving the potential of digital technology:

- Bottom-up approaches – people at the ground level who have innovative ideas need the support and resources to develop and implement new technology.
- Involving users in system design – digital technology can promote independent living. Users of the system, their family,

carers, health professionals and the public more generally, need to know how the system works – e.g., how it can help people with long-term conditions.

- Specific realistic goals and evaluation – evaluation is important for evidence-based decision making, e.g. measuring the immediate impact on users and health professionals should be the first priority, above the wider impact on services and their cost-effectiveness.

Web 2.0 technologies create a new landscape for health communication. There are different forms and functions of social media platforms. It is important to understand what is involved and what developers need to think about when developing social media platforms for health promotion activities. Keitzmann et al. (2011: 243) presented the 'social media ecology', a honeycomb framework of seven building blocks as a model for social media platforms. It showed the different functionalities, and their implications for the use of social media by organizations including healthcare. The seven building blocks are:

- Identity: the extent to which users reveal themselves,
- Conversations: the extent to which users communicate with each other,
- Sharing: the extent to which users exchange, distribute, and receive content,
- Presence: the extent to which users know if others are available,
- Relationships: the extent to which users relate to each other,
- Reputation: the extent to which users know the social standing of others and content,
- Groups: the extent to which users are ordered or form communities.

In order for social media site developers to develop strategies to maintain the validity and reliability of their social media platforms or applications, this honeycombed framework can be used as a tool to help with understanding their functionalities and implications when they are used for health communication. Keitzmann et al. (2011) also presented a guideline, the 4Cs, to help organizations in developing strategies for monitoring, understanding and responding to different social media activities. These are:

1 Cognize: recognize and understand the social media landscape;
2 Congruent: develop strategies that are congruent with different social media functionalities and goals of the organization;
3 Curate: act as a curator of social media interactions and content; and
4 Chase: a constant chase for information to understand the velocity of conversation flow and understand what is happening in the market, helping monitoring and evaluation.

Chou et al.'s (2013) study showed that social media are not consistent in following clinical guidelines or scientific evidence, which raises concerns on the credibility and accuracy of health information. Chou et al. proposed a similar process to Keitzmann et al.'s 4Cs guideline, to help to enhance the development of health promotion activities. They proposed the use of 'The STAR health promotion eHealth model' by Skinner et al. (2006), because of its emphasis on engagement and interactions with internet users, important in health promotion. The model involves five cycles of development:

1 identifying and understanding users' needs;
2 planning ways that technology can meet these needs;
3 implementing these plans in system design;
4 reviewing the system and adjusting the design based on user feedback; and
5 implementing the system.

These are useful models and processes for helping web developers in designing effective eHealth promotion interventions. As discussed in chapters 3 and 4, there are many social determinants influencing health, both within ourselves (such as our lifestyle, health literacy and digital skills, our motivation and self-efficacy (Bandura 1977) and our sense of coherence (Antonovsky 1996)), and externally in the immediate environment (such as social network and support, living and working conditions, health services) and the wider environment (such as the social, economic and cultural environment, as shown in the Dahlgren–Whitehead model (1991) and the social model of health). Chou et al. (2013) found that the majority of interventions do not encourage public participation and do not align to the principles and practice of health promotion. In the promotion of health, we need to take into account our understanding of what being healthy means to us, feeling empowered to participate within a supporting and enabling environment where the focus is on health rather than disease, as shown in the Salutogenic model of health (Antonovsky 1996).

The debate over digital technologies in widening digital divides has been ongoing over the last ten years. Some argued that the increased use of digital technologies enhances individual empowerment and participation in self-management of health, but others felt that the lack of access and low digital skills of some population groups will actually increase health inequality and inequity (Lee et al. 2014). As discussed in chapter 6, the digital divide is a cause for concern as it contributes to the worsening of health inequality and health inequity. With the ever-increasing functionality and complexity of innovative technologies and applications, improved health literacy and digital skills are essential for those with low digital literacy and low health literacy to ensure health equity. Lee et al. (2014) found that smartphones influence the digital divide and aggravate the gaps in terms of demographic access and digital skills. Accessibility has more of an impact on information, communication, leisure and financial management activities, followed by skills and the demographic gap. Their study showed that, although internet access has been improving globally, the debate now is about digital skills, usage and creative sharing. As the digital revolution progresses, the skills needed to participate in cyberspace are increasing and they shape effective online activities. So, although the gap resulting from socioeconomic status may decline, the gaps in internet usage and communication competence may greatly increase. Disengagement from smartphone use by people with low digital skills could lead to social, cultural and economic exclusion (Lee et al. 2014).

Chou et al. (2013) found that social media have not reduced digital divides and information disparities, and that there is not sufficient evidence that social media can reduce disparities or any problems relating to digital divides, although there are convincing data showing that some accessibility and access barriers are improving. Enabling equitable internet access for poor and rural populations remains a high priority. Our position defines our action in the achievement of health goals. An upstream approach to health, in which the structural factors are being addressed, is important in providing a supportive environment. Healthy public policies are also instrumental. Meaning and context, too, are important aspects determining how one behaves. A focus on health-orientated culture, the social practice where there is more freedom for understanding human behaviour, is more useful than targeting individual behaviours (Mielewczyk and Willig 2007; Cohn 2014). A behaviour approach (focusing solely on lifestyle interventions in a neoliberal climate where the focus is on the individual and the free market, and not on the wider structural environment) would have little effect, no matter how advanced the technologies are. The five action areas and the three strategies of health promotion – enable, mediate and advocate – encapsulating health promotion as discussed in the Ottawa Charter, remain relevant in our technologically advanced society (WHO 1986).

Digital health research practice

The interactive features of Web 2.0 and the vast amount of readily available data gathered in cyberspace are valuable in research, e.g. in health needs assessment exercises and evaluation of services provision. The Big Data phenomenon, as discussed in chapter 5, is important for public health management as well as for public health research. Data can be mined, analysed, repackaged and repurposed speedily. The surveillance and monitoring ability of internet applications is very useful in conducting good-quality research and improving healthcare. But the data-sharing features of Big Data can also cause concerns about data security and confidentiality, as discussed in chapter 5.

Research in eHealth is needed to assess its economic benefits and impact on population health (Piette et al. 2012). While evaluations of the role of eHealth are becoming more common, given the explosion in mobile phone usage alone, its impact remains difficult to measure (Keeton 2012). Chou et al. (2013) suggested several key themes and directions for research and practice related to the use of Web 2.0 social media platforms. There is a need to harness the participatory nature of social media. They suggested that future research in the use of Web 2.0 technologies should look at intervention feasibility and usability to ensure communication and the reach of health messages to a wider audience and improve the sustainability and engagement of target groups. With the interactiveness of Web 2.0 technology, the promotion of genuine participatory approaches is not just about consultation, it is an important aspect of working together throughout the whole research process, ensuring co-production does happen.

Innovative assessment methods are also needed for measuring dissemination, exposure engagement and effectiveness, illustrating the reach, impact and effect of health messages. Dynamic intervention design and implementation are needed for research (e.g. digital stories). Traditional study designs, such as randomized control trials and longitudinal cohort studies (even though claimed as the gold standard in some areas of health sciences) are not always methodologically sound at this stage for studying modern technologies. Partly this is because we are still at the early days of forming meaningful and robust research questions and how these can be answered. Methodology is contextual to the research process. Partly it is because language and meanings in this area are highly contested between different disciplines and paradigms. With the comprehensiveness of the Big Data phenomenon, techniques such as social network analysis can be used to better understand the complex interactions across users and platforms. Data mining and cloud-based computing techniques can be used to monitor and analyse social media content quantitatively and qualitatively. Validated machine learning models can also be used to assess patterns of social media content (Chou et al. 2013).

In general, eHealth is often technology-driven. Van Gemert-Pijnen et al. (2012) suggested that we need to address policy barriers and integrate traditional healthcare delivery with care that is enhanced by the use of technology. Policy makers and funders must promote, legislate and fund programmes and interventions that integrate and build upon a common m-health framework (Van Heerden et al. 2012). EHealth development must be holistic, evidence-based and people-centred, taking into account how people live (Van Gemert-Pijnen et al. 2012). Training and education in eHealth need to be included in medical and nursing training, as well as for all health-related and public health practitioners, to ensure professionals have the skills and abilities to incorporate and use modern technology in their work environment. Education is also needed for the general public so that they have the skills to access and use internet applications. It is also important to collaborate internationally to evaluate the impacts of eHealth. Van Heerden et al. suggested seven recommendations that are important to consider in mHealth research:

1 the need to develop evidence-based practice;
2 mHealth systems should be interoperable with existing eHealth initiatives;
3 mHealth should follow the same standards as for eHealth, which was designed for interoperability of health data and IT systems;
4 it should take a participatory approach;
5 a need to promote equity in health;
6 a need for sustainability of programmes;
7 a need to focus on health rather than on technology.

Web 3.0 era and the Internet of Things

As the development of new technology continues, we are arguably already in the Web 3.0 era: the Semantic Web, a smarter web that knows your personal profile and knows what you want to see. The participatory nature of Web 2.0 was a revolution after Web 1.0 technology. Its search ability is based on keywords and information is unorganized, whereas Web 3.0 technology enables computers to communicate with each other, objects to objects, so they are able to perform necessary tasks. This technology can understand the context of the user and provide useful information like an artificial intelligence (AI). Web 3.0 applications gather information, importing mined data and organizing it meaningfully, e.g. collecting data and providing warnings about natural disasters and new diseases (Aziz and Madani 2015). As we enter into this Web 3.0 era with the development of the Internet of Things (IoT), we are becoming part of the internet-connected network. The possibility of ever-changing and sophisticated healthcare applications is unimaginable. IoT allows machine-to-machine communication seamlessly among interconnected smarter physical objects within a cyberphysical infrastructure, without the need for human input. It has opened up many possibilities for healthcare, from enhancing health services and supporting independent living through smart homes and ambient assisted living, to the internet of mHealth; wearable body sensors for monitoring bodily functions and activating any medical interventions; tracking daily activities to provide suggestions for health improvements; and applications such as glucose-level monitoring; temperature, heart rate and blood pressure monitoring; medication monitoring, etc., and executing the appropriate actions.

Reducing costs of healthcare while improving health outcomes is a priority for policy makers. Neuhauser et al. (2013), studying the use of design science and AI to improve health communication, suggested that eHealth communication can improve traditional health communication through interactive personalized AI technology. Using sophisticated AI, health messages can be made personal, social and contextual for specific individuals, customized to individual health needs – e.g. avatars can be personal virtual health coaches, mimicking or enhancing human reasoning and behaviour, assessing multiple health variables in real time, automatically triggering support and information for specific individuals. However, most eHealth communication interventions have shown only modest results. AI technology is still in its infancy. More theoretically guided, interactive, culturally and psychologically engaging approaches, connecting to people's social contexts, are needed. Participatory user-centred design (from design to evaluation) is important – maybe even user-led or user-controlled. Could current systems and power relationships imagine such a reframing of power relationships? Over and above this, significant investment is also needed.

The IoT is about the interconnection of smarter objects, interlinking the physical world with the cyber world. Everyday objects may integrate intelligence and have the ability to sense, interpret and react to their environment. IoT enables people and things to be connected not only anytime, anywhere, but with anyone and anything, as well as any network and any service (Borgia 2014). However, its interoperability does posit risks to data security, such as cyberattack, privacy loss, confidentiality issues – particularly in these early days of development, where there is a lack of adoption of adequate standards (Miorandi et al. 2012; Tarouco et al. 2012; Santos et al. 2014; Islam et al. 2015). Although there are eHealth policies in many countries, many challenges exist

– e.g. standardization of interfaces and protocols across devices, customized computer platforms, resource limitations, app development, technology transition, quality of services, data security, human mobility, software compatibility, etc. Islam et al. (2015) proposed an intelligent security model that provides *protection* services to reduce cyberattacks, *detection* services to detect anomalies, and *reactive* services to defend against attacks. Data security remains the main challenge to date (Kouicem 2018). A collaborative approach among all stakeholders is needed at the global level as technologies develop into the future.

Final comments

Digital media have been used widely in health promotion, particularly in behaviour change campaigns such as the ones tackling smoking, drug use, sexual health and mental health. However, meaningful and rigorous evaluation is limited. Most studies on digital behaviour change campaigns show that they do not achieve behaviour change (Burke-Garcia and Scally 2014). The use of digital media is common. However, there is little evidence to show health community use in an effective manner. Burke-Garcia and Scally (2014) felt that the full potential of using digital media has not yet been achieved. They suggested that there are ten current trends of social media usage:

1   buzz monitoring and social research, which is an untapped area for the health sector;
2   Sharing of information and experience online bringing provider, researcher and consumer together;
3   information dissemination;
4   innovative partnership working allowing dissemination and sharing of health information to a larger but also highly targeted audience;
5   understanding the audiences so that the right message can get to the right audience;
6   use of health apps to help people with their own health improvement;
7   accessing health information anywhere with mobile technology;

8   need for rigorous and consistent measurement of data, and learning to manage Big Data;
9   involvement of senior leadership in digital communication; and
10 use of digital media for health campaigns.

Digital technology is changing the nature of health communication from traditional methods to digital methods, and from one way to two-way communication anytime, anywhere – and rapidly. Technologies offer many opportunities not only to disseminate, but also to gather information, allowing people to communicate, analyse, debate and understand health in new ways. Burke-Garcia and Scally (2014) argued for a new style of leadership, confident in digital communication such as Twitter. With better-informed programme planning, better information services, deeper relationship building, personalized health issues, technology building, more robust and meaningful measurement and evaluation, digital media could become the driver for health changes.

In a short space of twenty years, we have jumped from Web 1.0 information provision to the interactive Web 2.0 era, quickly arriving at the Web 3.0 and the Internet of Things era before even understanding the full potential of Web 2.0 technologies. As shown throughout this book, we are still learning how to harness the opportunities and possibilities of Web 2.0 technologies, digitizing health services and using them to maximize the potential for health communication, and developing evaluation methods to study their impact in the improvement of quality, effectiveness and efficiency of health services and health outcomes. Yet we are also leaping into innovative development such as the Internet of Things, developing applications unimaginable twenty years ago. In all of these innovations, strong leadership, exploration and healthy public policies are needed to manage this complex digital era in a fluid environment to ensure health and social equity. An empowering and enabling approach is also important in the promotion of good health and reducing health inequalities.

To draw a conclusion to this book, I will close with a list of recommendations:

1 Ensure the use of new technology is people-centred.
2 Collaborative approaches to working are needed, with policy

makers, web developers, health service managers, practitioners, researchers and the public involved in all aspects of development – strategically and technically, as well as in implementing and evaluating evidence-based practice.

3 A renewed focus on the social determinants of health is called for. This is, in part, about governments and policy makers paying more than lip service. It is also about presenting an alternative to neoliberal narratives in policy making and in the media. There need to be new stories about changing the world so that people are not left behind, rather than lurid stories about poverty, benefits fraud and fat-shaming. We need more system-changing and much less victim-blaming.

4 Adequate funding and investment – for development of new technologies; for research and evaluation of short-, medium- and long-term impacts on technology applications and interventions, as well as funding for education and training for people who use the technologies, including the public.

5 Effective leadership with adaptive change that ensures the engagement of health professionals and the public, who are the users of technology, with support necessary for implementation of new technology.

6 Harness the interoperability and integrating technologies into the wider system beyond healthcare, and develop strategies that focus on the structural factors that influence health; consider how technologies can help in the upstream approaches to healthcare;

7 Work with lifestyle-related industries to encourage a healthy culture where healthy choices are available and are the norm. Give people some empowering solutions.

8 Ensure policies and standards are in place for data security and data-sharing management in a connected world in the context of Big Data, so that there is confidence among all digital health users.

References

Acheson, D. (1998) *Independent Inquiry into Inequalities in Health Report*. London: Department of Health.

Agency for Healthcare Research and Quality (2011) *2010 National Healthcare Disparities and Quality Report (No. 11-0005)*. Rockville, MD: US Department of Health and Human Services.

Ahmad, F., Hudak, P. L., Bercovitz, K., Hollenberg, E. and Levinson, W. (2006) Are physicians ready for patients with Internet-based health information? *Journal of Medical Internet Research*, 8(3)e22:1–8.

Ajzen, I. (1991) The theory of planned behaviour. *Organisational Behaviour and Human Decision Processes*, 50:179–211.

Ajzen, I. and Fishbein, M. (1980) *Understanding Attitudes and Predicting Social Behaviour*. Englewood Cliffs, NJ: Prentice-Hall.

Akar, F. (2017) School Psychological Counsellors' opinions about causes and consequences of cyber bullying and preventive policies at schools. In *Multidisciplinary Academic Conference, AC-ETel 2017*. Prague: MAC Prague Consulting s.r.o.

Albu, M., Atack, L. and Srivastava, I. (2015) Simulation and gaming to promote health education: results of a usability test. *Health Education Journal*, 74(2):244–54.

Alghamdi, M., Gashgari, H. and Househ, M. (2015) A systematic review of mobile health technology use in developing countries. *Studies in Health Technology Informatics*, 213:223–6.

Andreasen, A. R. (1995) *Marketing Social Change: Changing Behaviour to Promote Health, Social, Development, and the Environment*. San Francisco: Jossey-Bass Publications.

Andreasen, A. R. (2003) The life trajectory of social marketing. *Marketing Theory*, 3(3):293–304.

Antonovsky, A. (1979) *Health, Stress and Coping*. San Francisco: Jossey-Bass Publications.

Antonovsky, A. (1987) *Unravelling the Mystery of Health*. San Francisco: Jossey-Bass Publications.

Antonovsky, A. (1996) The Salutogenic model as a theory to guide health promotion. *Health Promotion International*, 11(1):11–18.

Atkin, C. K. and Rice, R. E. (2013) Advances in public communication campaigns. In E. Scharrer (ed.) *The International Encyclopaedia of Media Studies*, Vol. V: *Media Effects / Media Psychology*. London: Wiley-Blackwell.

Atkin, C. K. and Salmon, C. (2010) Communication campaigns. In C. Berger, M. Roloff and D. Roskos-Ewoldsen (eds.) *Handbook of Communication Sciences* (2nd edn.). Thousand Oaks, CA: Sage.

Ayo, N. (2010) Understanding health promotion in a neoliberal climate and the making of health-conscious citizens. *Critical Public Health*, 22(1):99–105.

Aziz, H. A. and Madani, A. (2015) Evolution of the Web and its uses in healthcare. *Clinical Laboratory Science*, 28(4):245–9.

Baggott, R. (2015) *Understanding Health Policy* (2nd edn). Bristol: Policy Press.

Baig, M. M., Gholam-Hosseini, H. and Connolly, M. J. (2015) Mobile healthcare applications: system design review, critical issues and challenges. *Australasian College of Physical Scientists and Engineers in Medicine*, 38:23–38.

Bailey, J., Mann, S., Wayal, S., et al. (2015) Sexual health promotion for young people delivered via digital media: a scoping review. *Public Health Research*, 3(13).

Bandura, A. (1977) Self-efficacy: toward a unifying theory of behavioural change. *Psychological Review*, 84:191–215.

Bandura, A. (2004) Health promotion by social cognitive means. *Health Education and Behaviour*, 31(2):143–64.

Baric, L. (1994) *Health Promotion and Health Education in*

Practice. Module 2: The Organisational Model. Altrincham: Barns Publications.

Barrett, M. and Gershkovich, M. (2013) Computers and psychotherapy: are we out of a job? *Psychotherapy*, 51(2):220–3.

Barrett, M., Humblet, O., Hiatt, R. and Adler, N. (2013) Big data and disease prevention: from quantified self to quantified communities. *Big Data*, 1:168–75.

Baum, F. and Fisher, M. (2014) Why behavioural health promotion endures despite its failure to reduce health inequities. *Sociology of Health and Illness*, 36(2):213–25.

Baum, F., Newman, L. and Biedrzycki, K. (2012) Vicious cycles: digital technologies and determinants of health in Australia. *Health Promotion International*, 29(2):349–60.

Beattie, A. (1991) Knowledge and control in health promotion: a test case for social policy. In J. Gabe, M. Calnan and M. Bury (eds.) *The Sociology of the Health Service*. London: Routledge and Kegan Paul.

Beauchamp, T. L. and Childress, J. F. (1994) *Principles of Biomedical Ethics*. New York: Oxford University Press.

Becker, M. H. (ed.) (1984) *The Health Belief Model and Personal Health Behavior*. Thorofare, NJ: Charles B. Slack.

Becker, C. M., Glascoff, M. A. and Felts, W.M. (2010) Salutogenesis 30 years later: where do we go from here? *International Electronic Journal of Health Education*, 13:25–32.

Bennett, G. G. and Glasgow, R. E. (2009) The delivery of public health interventions via the Internet: actualizing their potential. *Annual Review Public Health*, 30:273–92.

Beresford, P., Fleming, J., Glynn, M., et al. (2011) *Supporting People*. Bristol: Policy Press.

Berg, M., Mattinen, H. and Pattugalan, G. (2013) *Examining Protection and Gender in Cash and Voucher Transfers*. Rome: World Food Programme and The United Nations Refugee Agency.

Berkman, N. D., Davis, T. C. and McCormack, L. (2010) Health literacy: what is it? *Journal of Health Communication*, 15:9–19.

Bert, F., Giacometti, M., Gualano, M. R. and Siliquini, R. (2014) Smartphones and health promotion: a review of the evidence. *Journal of Medical Systems*, 38(1):9995.

Bhuyan, S. S., Kim, H., Isehunwa, O. O., et al. (2017) Privacy and security issues in mobile health: current research and future directions. *Health Policy and Technology*, 6:188–91.

References

Bhuyan, S. S., Lu, N., Chandak, A., et al. (2016) Use of mobile health applications for health-seeking behaviour among US adults. *Journal of Medical Systems*, 40:153.

Birnbaum, F., Lewis, D., Rosen, R. K. and Ranney, M. L. (2015) Patient engagement and the design of digital health. *Academic Emergency Medicine*, 22(6):754–6.

Bisoglio, J., Michaels, T. I., Mervis, J. E. and Ashinoff, B. K. (2014) Cognitive enhancement through action video game training: great expectations. *Frontiers in Psychology*, 5(136):1–9.

Black, A. D., Car, J., Pagliari, C., et al. (2011) The impact of eHealth on the quality and safety of health care: a systematic overview. *PLoS Medicine*, 18:8(1):e1000387.

Blades, M. Oates, C. and Li, S. (2013) Children's recognition of advertisements on television and on Web pages. *Appetite*, 62:190–3.

Bloomfield, G. S., Vedanthan, R., Vasudevan, L., Kithei, A., Were, M. and Velazquez, E. J. (2014) Mobile health for non-communicable diseases in Sub-Saharan Africa: a systematic review of the literature and strategic framework for research. *Globalisation and Health*, 10:49.

Boehm, A. and Staples, L.H. (2004). Empowerment: the point of view of consumers. *Families in Society*, 85(2):270–80.

Boelsen-Robinson, T., Backholer, K. and Peeters, A. (2015) Digital marketing of unhealthy foods to Australian children and adolescents. *Health Promotion International*, 31:523–53.

Borgia, E. (2014) The Internet of Things vision: key features, applications and open issues. *Computer Communications*, 54:1–31.

Bossewitch, J. and Sinnreich, A. (2013) The end of forgetting: strategic agency beyond the panopticon. *New Media and Society*, 15(2):224–42.

Boulos, M. N. K., Gammon, S., Dixon, M. C., et al. (2015) Digital games for type 1 and type 2 diabetes: underpinning theory with three illustrative examples. *Journal of Medical Internet Research*, 3(1):e3.

Boulos, M. N. K. and Yang, S. (2013) Exergames for health and fitness: the roles of GPS and geosocial apps. *International Journal of Health Geographics*, 12(18):1–7.

Bowen, E., Walker, K., Mawer, M., Holdsworth, E., Sorbring, E. and Helsing, B. (2014) 'It's like you're actually playing as yourself': development and preliminary evaluation of 'Green Acres High'. *Psychosocial Intervention*, 23:43–55.

Braa, J., Heywood, A. and Sahay, S. (2012) Improving quality and use of data through data-use workshops: Zanzibar, United Republic of Tanzania. *Bulletin of the World Health Organization*, 90:379–84.

Brusse, C., Gardner, K., McAullay, D. and Dowden, M. (2014) Social media and mobile apps for health promotion in Australian Indigenous populations: scoping review. *Journal of Medical Internet Research*, 16(12):e280.

Buck, D. and Maguire, D. (2015) *Inequalities in Life Expectancy: Changes Over Time and Implications for Policy*. London: The King's Fund.

Burke-Garcia, A. and Scally, G. (2014) Trending now: future directions in digital media for the public health sector. *Journal of Public Health*, 36(4):527–34.

Campbell, J. L., Fletcher, E., Britten, N., et al. (2014) Telephone triage for management of same-day consultation requests in general practice (the ESTEEM trial): a cluster-randomised controlled trial and cost consequence analysis. *Lancet*, 384(9957):1859–68.

Capurro, D., Cole, K., Echavarría, M. I., Joe, J., Neogi, T. and Turner, A. M. (2014) The use of social networking sites for public health practice and research: a systematic review. *Journal of Medical Internet Research*, 16(3):e79.

Carter, S. M., Cribb, A. and Allegrante, J. P. (2012) How to think about health promotion ethics. *Public Health Reviews*, 34(1):1–24.

Castells, M. (2011) A network theory of power. *International Journal of Communication*, 5:773–787.

Cavallo, D. N., Tate, D. F., Ries, A. V., Brown, J. D., DeVellis, R. F. and Ammerman, A. S. (2012) A social media-based physical activity intervention. *American Journal of Preventive Medicine*, 43(5):527–32.

Centers for Disease Control and Prevention (CDC) (2017) *Childhood Obesity Facts* [online]. Centers for Disease Control and Prevention, US Department of Health and Human Services. Available at: www.cdc.gov/healthyschools/obesity/facts.htm.

Centre for Health Promotion, Women's and Children's Health Network (2012) *Where They Hang Out: Social Media Use in*

Youth Health Promotion. Adelaide: Department of Health, Government of South Australia.

Chen, W. H. (2013) The implications of social capital for the digital divides in America. *Information Society*, 29:13–25.

Chesser, A., Burke, A., Reyes, J. and Rohrberg, T. (2015) Navigating the digital divide: a systematic review of eHealth literacy in underserved populations in the United States. *Informatics for Health and Social Care*, 41(1):1–19.

Chib, A., van Velthoven, M. H. and Car, J. (2014) mHealth adoption in low-resource environments: a review of the use of mobile healthcare in developing countries. *Journal of Health Communication*, 20(1):4–34.

Choi, N. G. and DiNitto, D. M. (2013) The Digital Divide among low-income homebound older adults: Internet use patterns, eHealth literacy, and attitudes toward computer/internet use. *Journal of Medical Internet Research*, 15(5):e93.

Chou, W. Y. S., Prestin, A., Lyons, C. and Wen, K. Y. (2013) Web 2.0 for health promotion: reviewing the current evidence. *American Journal of Public Health*, 103:E9–E11.

Chriss, J. J. (2015) Nudging and social marketing. *Social Science and Public Policy*, 52:54–61.

Clampitt, P. (2001) *Communicating for Managerial Effectiveness* (2nd edn). Thousand Oaks, CA: Sage.

C4CC (Coalition for Collaborative Care) (2014) *A Co-production Model*. Leeds: NHS England and Coalition for Collaborative Care.

Cohn, S. (2014) From health behaviours to health practices: an introduction. *Sociology of Health and Illness*, 36(2):157–62.

Coiera, E. (2013) Social networks, social media, and social diseases. *British Medical Journal*, 346:f3007.

Coleman, C., Kurtz-Rossi, S., McKinney, J., Pleasant, A., Rootman, I. and Shohet, L. (2011) *Calgary Charter on Health Literacy*. Quebec: The Centre for Literacy.

Coleman, C. A., Nguyen, N. T., Garvin, R., Sou, C. and Carney, P. A. (2016) Health literacy teaching in US family medicine residency programs: a national survey. *Journal of Health Communication*, 21:sup.1:51–7.

Commission on Social Determinants of Health (CSDH) (2008). *Closing the Gap in a Generation: Health Equity Through Action on the Social Determinants of Health. Final Report of the Commission on Social Determinants of Health.* Geneva: World Health Organization.

Concepcion, H. (2017) Video game therapy as an intervention for children with disabilities. *Therapeutic Recreation Journal*, L1(3):221–8.

Conner, M. and Norman, P. (eds.) (2015) *Predicting and Changing Health Behaviour: Research and Practice with Social Cognition Models* (3rd edn). Maidenhead: Open University Press.

COPPA (1998) The Children's Online Privacy Protection Act 1998. US Government Publishing Office.

Coulter, A. and Mearns, B. (2016) *Developing Care for a Changing Population: Patient Engagement and Health Information Technology*. London: Nuffield Trust.

Council of Europe (2011) *Council of Europe Convention on Preventing and Combating Violence against Women and Domestic Violence*. Council of Europe Treaty Series, 210. Istanbul: Council of Europe.

Crawford, R. (1980) Healthism and the medicalisation of everyday life. *International Journal of Health Services*, 10(3):365–88.

Crawshaw, P. (2013) Public health policy and the behavioural turn: the case of social marketing. *Critical Social Policy*, 33:616–37.

Cribb, A. and Duncan, P. (2002) *Health Promotion and Professional Ethics*. Oxford: Blackwell.

Cross, R., Davis, S. and O'Neil, I. (2017) *Health Communication: Theoretical and Critical Perspectives*. Cambridge: Polity.

Dahlgren, G. and Whitehead, M. (1991) *Policies and Strategies to Promote Social Equity in Health*. Stockholm: Institute of Future Studies.

Davies, A., Keeble, E., Bhatia, T. and Fisher, E. (2016) *Public Health and Prevention*. QualityWatch. London: The Health Foundation and Nuffield Trust.

Dean, M. (1999) *Governmentality: Power and Rule in Modern Society*. London: Sage.

Deloitte Centre for Health Solutions (2015) *Connected Health: How Digital Technology Is Transforming Health and Social Care*. London: The Creative Studio at Deloitte.

DeMartini, T. L., Beck, A. F., Klein, M. D. and Kahn, R. S. (2013) Access to digital technology among families coming to urban paediatric primary care clinics. *Paediatrics*, 132(1)e142–e148.

Dennison, L., Morrison, L., Conway, G. and Yardley, L. (2013)

Opportunities and challenges for smartphone applications in supporting health behavior change: qualitative study. *Journal of Medical Internet Research*, 15:e86.

Department of Health (DH) (1992) *The Health of the Nation: A Strategy for Health*. London: HMSO.

Department of Health (DH) (1999) *Saving Lives: Our Healthier Nation*. London: HMSO.

Department of Health (DH) (2004) *Choosing Health: Making Healthier Choices Easier*. London: HMSO.

Department of Health (DH) (2010a) *Improving the Health and Well-being of People with Long-term Conditions*. London: HMSO.

Department of Health (DH) (2010b) *Equity and Excellence: Liberating the NHS Report*. London: HMSO.

Department of Health (DH) (2012a) *Digital Strategy Report*. London: HMSO.

Department of Health (DH) (2012b) *The Power of Information*. London: HMSO.

Department of Health (DH) (2012c) *Long-term Conditions Compendium of Information* (3rd edn). Available at www.dh.gov.uk/publications

Department of Health (DH) (2013a) *Statutory Guidance on Joint Strategic Needs Assessment and Joint Health and Wellbeing*. London: HMSO.

Department of Health (DH) (2013b) *The Digital Challenge: How a Paperless NHS Will Improve Services*. London: HMSO.

Department of Health and Social Security (DHSS) (1980) *Inequalities in Health: Report of a Research Working Group*. London: Department of Health and Social Security.

Dewey, J. (1916) *Democracy and Education*. New York: Macmillan. Cited in S. D. Brookfield and S. Preskill (1999) *Discussion as a Way of Teaching – Tools and Techniques for University Teachers*. London: The Society for Research into Higher Education, and Open University Press.

Dibb, S. (2014) Up, up and away: social marketing breaks free. *Journal of Marketing Management*, 30(11–12):1159–85.

Dixey, R. (ed.) (2013) *Health Promotion: Global Principles and Practice*. Oxford: CABI.

Dooris, M. (2005) Healthy settings: challenges to generating evidence of effectiveness. *Health Promotion International,* 21:55–65.

Dredze, M. (2012) How social media will change public health. *IEEE Intelligent Systems,* 27:81–4.

Duggan, M. and Brenner, J. (2013) *The Demographics of Social Media Users – 2012.* Washington, DC: The Pew Internet and American Life Project.

Ennis, L., Rose, D., Denis, M., Pandit, N. and Wykes, T. (2012) Can't surf, won't surf: the digital divide in mental health. *Journal of Mental Health,* 21(4):395–403.

Ephraim, P. E. (2013) African youths and the dangers of social networking: a culture-centred approach to using social media. *Ethics Information Technology,* 15: 275–84.

Eriksson, M. and Lindstrom, B. (2008) A salutogenic interpretation of the Ottawa Charter. *Health Promotion International,* 23:190–9.

Espie, C. A., Kyle, S. D., Williams, C., et al. (2012) A randomized, placebo-controlled trial of online cognitive behavioural therapy for chronic insomnia disorder delivered via an automated media-rich web application. *Sleep,* 35(6)769–781B.

Estcourt, C. S., Gibbs, J., Sutcliffe, L. J., et al. (2017) The eSexual health clinic system for management, prevention, and control of sexually transmitted infections: exploratory studies in people testing for Chlamydia trachomatis. *Lancet Public Health,* 2:182–90.

Etkin, J. (2016) The hidden cost of personal quantification. *Journal of Consumer Research,* 42:967–84.

European Commission (2012) eHealth Action Plan 2012–2020 – innovative healthcare for the 21st century. Brussels: European Commission.

European Health Literacy Consortium (2012) *Comparative Report on Health Literacy in Eight EU Member States: The European Health Literacy Project 2009–2012.* Maastricht: HLS-EU Consortium.

The Evidence Centre (2014) *Does Health Coaching Work?* Cambridge: Health Education East of England.

Farnell, G. and Barkley, J. (2017) The effect of a wearable physical activity monitor (Fitbit One) on physical activity behaviour in women: a pilot study. *Journal of Human Sport and Exercise,* 12(4):1230–7.

Federal Trade Commission (2006) Federal Trade Commission Act Incorporating U.S. SAFE WEB Act Amendments of 2006. Washington, DC: US Government Publishing Office.

Fernández-Aranda, F., Jiménez-Murcia, S., Santamaría, J. J., et al. (2012) Video games as a complementary therapy tool in mental disorders: PlayMancer, a European multicentre study. *Journal of Mental Health*, 21(4):364–74.

Fletcher, S. and Mullett, J. (2016) Digital stories as a tool for health promotion and youth engagement. *Canadian Journal of Public Health*, 107(2):e183–7.

Food Foundation (2017) *UK's Restrictions on Junk Food Advertising to Children*. London: The Food Foundation.

Foucault, M., (1979) Governmentality. *Ideology and Consciousness*, 6:5–21.

Fox, S. and Duggan, M. (2012) *Mobile Health Report*. Washington, DC: Pew Research Centre.

Fox, S. and Jones, S. (2009) *The Social Life of Health Information*. Washington, DC: Pew Internet and American Life Project.

Free, C., Phillips, G., Galli, L., et al. (2013) The effectiveness of mobile-health technology-based health behaviour change or disease management interventions for health care consumers: a systematic review. *PLOS Medicine*, 10(1):e1001362.

Freire, P. (1972) *Pedagogy of the Oppressed*. Harmondsworth: Penguin.

Freire, P. (1973). *Education for Critical Consciousness*. New York: Continuum Publishing Company.

Frohlich, K. L. and Abel, T. (2013) Environmental justice and health practices: understanding how health inequities arise at the local level. *Sociology of Health and Illness*, 36(2):199–212.

Gaventa, J. (2006) Finding the spaces for change: a power analysis. In R. Eyben, C. Harris and J. Pettit (eds.) Exploring Power for Change, *Institute of Development Studies Bulletin*, 37:6.

GDPR (2018) *EU General Data Protection Regulation (GDPR)*. Brussels: European Parliament and Council of the European Union.

Gibbons, M. C., Fleisher, L., Slamon, R. E., Bass, S., Kandadai, V. and Beck, J. R. (2011) Exploring the potential of Web 2.0 to address health disparities. *Journal of Health Communication*, 16(Sup.1):77–89.

Glasheen, K. J., Shochet, I. and Campbell, M. A. (2015) Online counselling in secondary schools: would students seek help by this medium? *British Journal of Guidance and Counselling*, 44(1):108–22.

Godfrey, A. (2017) Wearables for independent living in older adults: gait and falls. *Maturitas*, 100:16–26.

Gold, J., Pedrana, A. E., Sacks-Davis, R., et al. (2011) A systematic examination of the use of online social networking sites for sexual health promotion. *BioMed Central Public Health*, 11:583.

Gold, J., Pedrana, A. E., Stoove, M. A., et al. (2012) Developing health promotion interventions on social networking sites: recommendations from The Face Space Project. *Journal of Medical Internet Research*, 14(1):e30.

Good Things Foundation (2016) *Health and Digital: Reducing Inequalities, Improving Society: An Evaluation of the Widening Digital Participation Programme.* Sheffield: Good Things Foundation.

Goodwin, T. (2012) Why we should reject 'nudge'. *Politics*, 32(2):85–92.

Gordon, R., Russell-Bennett, R. and Lefebvre, R. C. (2016) Social marketing: the state of play and brokering the way forward. *Journal of Marketing Management*, 32(11–12):1059–82.

Gowin, M., Cheney, M., Gwin, S. and Wann, T. F. (2015) Health and fitness app use in college students: a qualitative study. *American Journal of Health Education*, 46:223–30.

Grady, A., Yoong, S., Sutherland, R., Lee, H., Nathan, N. and Wolfenden, L. (2018) Improving the public health impact of eHealth and mHealth interventions. *Australian and New Zealand Journal of Public Health*, 42(2):118–19.

Green, J., Tones, K., Cross, R. and Woodall, J. (2015) *Health Promotion: Planning and Strategies* (3rd edn). London: Sage.

Gregg, J. and O'Hara, L. (2007) Values and principles evident in current health promotion practice. *Health Promotion Journal Australia*, 18(1):7–11.

Gregoire, C. (2014) Why these neuroscientists are prescribing video games [online]. *The Huffington Post*. Available at: www.huffin gtonpost.co.uk/2014/10/29/autism-video-games_n_6056634.ht ml.

Gretton, C. and Honeyman, M. (2016) *The Digital Revolution: Eight Technologies That Will Change Health and Care*. London: The King's Fund.

Greysen, S. R., Kind, T. and Chretien, K. C. (2010) Online professionalism and the mirror of social media. *Society of General Internal Medicine*, 25(11):1227–9.

Grier, S. and Bryant, C. A. (2005) Social marketing in public health. *Annual Review of Public Health*, 26:319–39.

Guse, K., Levine, D., Martins, S., et al. (2012) Interventions using new digital media to improve adolescent sexual health: a systematic review. *Journal of Adolescent Health*, 51:535–43.

Guttman, N. (1995) Ethical dilemmas in health campaigns. Unpublished conference proceedings for the 1995 Annual Conference of the International Communication Association. Washington.

Guttman, N. (1997) Ethical dilemmas in health campaigns. *Health Communication*, 9(2):155–90.

Hampshire, K., Porter, G., Owusu, S. A., et al. (2015) Informal m-health: how are young people using mobile phones to bridge healthcare gaps in Sub-Saharan Africa? *Social Science and Medicine*, 142:90–9.

Hanson, C., Thackeray, R., Barnes, M., Neiger, B. and McIntyre, E. (2008) Integrating Web 2.0 in health education preparation and practice. *American Journal of Health Education*, 39(3):157–66.

Harrison, T. (2016) Virtuous reality: moral theory and research into cyber-bullying. *Ethics Information Technology*, 17:275–83.

Hazelwood, A. (2008) Using text messaging in the treatment of eating disorders. *Nursing Times*, 104(40):28–9.

He, D., Naveed, M., Gunter, C. A. and Nahrstedt, K. (2014) Security concerns in Android mHealth apps. *AMIA Annual Symposium Proceedings, American Medical Informatics Association* Symposium, 2014:645–54.

Head, K. J., Noar, S. M., Iannarino, N. T. and Harrington, N. G. (2013) Efficacy of text messaging-based interventions for health promotion: a meta-analysis. *Social Science and Medicine*, 97: 41–8.

Health on the Net Foundation (2013) *Health on the Net (HON) Code of Conduct for Medical and Health Web Sites*. Geneva: Health on the Net Foundation.

Herschel, R. and Miori, V. M. (2017) Ethics and Big Data. *Technology in Society*, 49:31–6.

Hill, S., Merchant, R. and Ungar, L. (2013) Lessons learned about public health from online crowd surveillance. *Big Data*, 1:160–7.

HM Government (2010) *Healthy Lives, Healthy People: Our Strategy for Public Health in England*. London: HMSO.

HM Government (2015) *Chancellor Announces £4½ Billions of Measures to Bring Down Debt*. London: HMSO. Available at www.gov.uk/government/news/chancellor-announces-4-billion-of-measures-to-bring-down-debt.

HM Treasury (2015) *Spending Review and Autumn Statement 2015*. London: HM Treasury.

Ho, J., Cordena, M. E., Caccamoa, L., et al. (2016) Design and evaluation of a peer network to support adherence to a web-based intervention for adolescents. *Internet Interventions*, 6:50–6.

Hoise, A., Vogl, G., Hoddinott, J., Carden, J. and Comeau, Y. (2014) *Crossroads: Rethinking the Australian Mental Health System*. Pyrmont: ReachOut.com by Inspire Foundation.

Honeyman, M., Dunn, P. and McKenna, H. (2016) *A Digital NHS? An Introduction to the Digital Agenda and Plans for Implementation*. London: The King's Fund.

Hopwood, T. and Merritt, R. (2011) *Big Pocket Guide to Using Social Marketing for Behaviour Change*. London: National Social Marketing Centre.

Horgan, A. and Sweeney, J. (2010) Young students' use of the internet for mental health information and support. *Journal of Psychiatric Mental Health Nursing*, 17(2):117–23.

Horne-Moyer, H. L., Moyer, B. H., Messer, D. C. and Messer, E. S. (2014) The use of electronic games in therapy: a review with clinical implications. *Current Psychiatry Report*, 16:520.

Horrocks, C. and Johnson, S. (2014) A socially situated approach to inform ways to improve health and wellbeing. *Sociology of Health and Illness*, 36(2):175–86.

Hou, J. and Shim, M. (2010) The role of provider–patient communication and trust in online sources in internet use for health-related activities. *Journal of Health Communication: International Perspectives*, 15(S3):186–99.

House of Commons Health Committee (2016) *Public Health Post-2013*. London: House of Commons.

Hsieh, R. L., Lee, W. C. and Lin, J. H. (2016). The impact of short-term video games on performance among children with developmental delays: a randomized controlled trial. *PLOS ONE*, 11(3):e0149714.

Hswen, Y., Brownstein, J. S., Liu, J. and Hawkins, J. B. (2017) Use of a digital health application for influenza surveillance in China. *American Journal of Public Health*, 107:1130–6.

Huber, M., Knottnerus, J. A., Green, L., et al. (2011) How should we define health? *British Medical Journal*, 343(7817):235–7.

Hubley, J. (2004) *Communicating Health: An Action Guide to Health Education and Health Promotion* (2nd edn). London: Macmillan Education.

Hubley, J. and Copeman, J. (2008) *Practical Health Promotion*. Cambridge: Polity.

Huckvale, K., Prieto, J. T., Tilney, M., Benghozi, P. and Car, J. (2015) Unaddressed privacy risks in accredited health and wellness apps: a cross-sectional systematic assessment. *BMC Medicine*, 13:214.

Hunjan, R. and Keophilavong, S. (2010) *Power and Making Change Happen*. Dunfermline: Carnegie UK Trust.

Hunt, J. (2013). Jeremy Hunt challenges NHS to go paperless by 2018 [online]. Press release, 16 January. Available at: www.gov.uk/government/news/jeremy-hunt-challenges-nhs-to-go-paperless-by-2018.

Hunter, R. F., Gough, A., Kane, N. O., et al. (2018) Ethical issues in social media research for public health. *American Journal of Public Health*, 108(3):343–8.

IMS Health (2015) *Availability and Profile of Consumer mHealth Apps*. NJ: IMS Institute for Healthcare Informatics.

Ipsos MORI (2015) *GP Patient Survey: National Summary Report*. Leeds: NHS England.

Islam, S. M. R., Kwak, D., Kabir, H., Hossain, M. and Kwak, K. (2015) The Internet of Things for health care: a comprehensive survey. *IEEE Access*, 10.1109.

iSMA (International Social Marketing Association), ESMA (European Social Marketing Association) and AASM (Australian Association of Social Marketing) (2013) *Consensus Definition of Social Marketing as Endorsed by iSMA, ESMA and AASM* [online]. Available at www.i-socialmarketing.org/assets/social_marketing_definition.pdf.

IUHPE (2016) *Core Competencies and Professional Standards for Health Promotion*. Paris: International Union for Health Promotion and Education.

IUHPE (2018) IUHPE position statement on Health Literacy: a practical vision for a health literate world. *Global Health Promotion*, 25(4):79–88.

Janz, N. K. and Becker, M. H. (1984) The Health Belief Model: a decade later. *Health Education Quarterly*, 11:1–47.

Javitt, J. (2014) *The Future in Hand: mHealth Technologies Hold Promise for Better Managing Chronic Illness*. Chicago: Healthcare Information and Management Systems Society (HIMSS).

Johnson, C. W. (2010) *Case Studies in the Failure of Healthcare Information Systems*. University of Glasgow, Department of Computing Science.

Jung, D. and Jeong, W. (2011) Nudge: a tool for better policy impacts and its limitations under various policy contexts. *Public Administration Review*, July/August 2011:653–6.

Karami, A., Dahl, A. A., Turner-McGrievy, G., Kharrazi, H. and Shaw, G. (2018) Characterizing diabetes, diet, exercise and obesity comments on Twitter. *International Journal of Information Management*, 38(1):1–6.

Karapanos, E., Gouveia, R., Hassenzahl, M. and Jodi Forlizzi, J. (2016) Wellbeing in the making: peoples' experiences with wearable activity trackers. *Psychology of Well-Being*, 6:4.

Keeton, C. (2012) Measuring the impact of eHealth. *Bulletin of the World Health Organization*, 90:326–7.

Keitzmann, J. H., Hermkens, K., McCarthy, I. P. and Silvestre, B. S. (2011) Social media? Get serious! Understanding the functional building blocks of social media. *Business Horizons*, 54:241–51.

Kelly, L., Ziebland, S. and Jenkinson, C. (2015) Measuring the effects of online health information: scale validation for the eHealth Impact questionnaire. *Patient Education and Counselling*, 98:1418–24.

Kemp, S. (2016) Digital in 2016 [online]. We Are Social website. Available at https://wearesocial.com/uk.

Kemp, S. (2018) Digital in 2018 [online]. We Are Social website. Available at https://wearesocial.com/uk.

Kitchin, R. and Lauriault, T. (2014) *Towards Critical Data Studies: Charting and Unpacking Data Assemblages and Their Work* [online]. The Programmable City Working Paper 2. Available at: www.researchgate.net/publication/267867447_Towards_critic al_data_studies_Charting_and_unpacking_data_assemblages_a nd_their_work.

Klasnja, P. and Pratt, W. (2012). Healthcare in the pocket: mapping the space of mobile-phone health interventions. *Journal of Biomedical Informatics*, 45(1):184–98.

Kohut, A., Wike, R., Horowitz, J. M., et al. (2011). *Global Digital Communication: Texting, Social Networking Popular Worldwide*. Washington, DC: Pew Global Attitudes Project.

Korda, H. and Itani, Z. (2013) Harnessing social media for health promotion and behaviour change. *Health Promotion Practice*, 14:15–23.

Kotler, P. and Levy, S. J. (1969) Broadening the concept of Marketing. *Journal of Marketing*, 33:10–15.

Kotler, P. and Zaltman, G. (1971) Social marketing: an approach to planned social change. *Journal of Marketing*, 35:3–12.

Kouicem, D. E., Bouabdallah, A. and Lakhlef, H. (2018) Internet of things security: a top-down survey. *Computer Networks*, 141:199–221.

Kramer, J. N. and Kowatsch, T. (2017) Using feedback to promote physical activity: the role of the feedback sign. *Journal of Medical Internet Research*, 19(6):e192.

Krebs, P. and Duncan, D. T. (2015) Health apps use among US mobile phone owners: a national survey. *Journal of Medical Internet Research, Mhealth Uhealth*, 3(4):101.

Kreuter, M. T. and McClure, S. M. (2004) The role of culture in health communication. *Annual Review Public Health*, 25:439–55.

Kwankam, S. Y. (2012) Successful partnerships for international collaboration in e-health: the need for organized national infrastructures. *Bulletin of the World Health Organization*, 90:332–40.

Lafferty, N. (2013) *NHS-HE Connectivity Project: Web 2.0 and Social Media in Education and Research*. Dundee: NHS-HE Connectivity Best Practice Working Group of the NHS-HE Forum.

Lalonde, M. (1974) *A New Perspective on the Health of Canadians*. Ottawa: Public Health Agency of Canada.

Lasswell, H. D. (1948) The structure and function of

communication in society. In D. McQuail and S. Windahl (1993) *Communication Models for the Study of Mass Communication* (2nd edn). London: Longman.

Laverack, G. (2009) *Public Health: Power, Empowerment and Professional Practice* (2nd edn). London: Palgrave Macmillan.

Laverack, G. (2013) *Health Activism: Foundations and Strategies*. London: Sage Publications.

Laverack, G. (2017) The challenge of behaviour change and health promotion. *Challenges*, 8(25): Commentary 1–4.

Lawrence, D., Johnson, S., Hafekost, J., et al. (2015) *The Mental Health of Children and Adolescents: Report on the Second Australian Child and Adolescent Survey of Health and Wellbeing*. Canberra: Australian Government.

Ledger, D. (2014) *Inside Wearables – Part 2*. Cambridge, MA: Endeavour Partners LLC.

Lee, H., Park, N. and Hwang, Y. (2014) A new dimension of the digital divide: exploring the relationship between broadband connection, smartphone use and communication competence. *Telematics and Informatics*, 32:45–56.

Lee, M. S., Wu, Z. P. Svanstrom, L. and Dalal, K. (2013) Cyber bullying prevention: intervention in Taiwan. *PLOS ONE*, 8(5):e64031.

Lefebvre, C. (2009) Integrating cell phones and mobile technologies into public health practice: a social marketing perspective. *Health Promotion Practice*, 10(4):490–4.

Lewis, T., Synowiec, C., Lagomarsinoa, G. and Schweitzera, J. (2012) E-health in low- and middle-income countries: findings from the Centre for Health Market Innovations. *Bulletin of the World Health Organization*, 90:332–340.

Lim, M. S. C., Wright, C. J. C., Carrotte, E. R. and Pedrana, A. E. (2016) Reach, engagement, and effectiveness: a systematic review of evaluation methodologies used in health promotion via social networking sites. *Health Promotion Journal of Australia*, 27:187–97.

Lindstrom, B. and Eriksson, M. (2010) A Salutogenic approach to tackling health inequalities. In A. Morgan, E. Ziglio and M. Davies (eds.) *Health Assets in a Global Context: Theory, Methods, Action*. New York, Dordrecht, Heidelberg, London: Springer.

Lister, C., West, J. H., Cannon, B., Sax, T. and Brodegard, D.

(2014) Just a fad? Gamification in health and fitness apps. *Journal of Medical Internet Research*, 2(2):e9.

Lorenc, T., Petticrew, M., Welch, V. and Tugwell, P. (2012) What types of interventions generate inequalities? Evidence from systematic reviews. *Journal of Epidemiology Community Health* jech-2012-201257.

Loss, J., Lindacher, V. and Curbach, J. (2014) Online social networking sites – a novel setting for health promotion? *Health and Place*, 26:161–70.

Lovell, S., Kearns, R. A. and Prince, R. (2014) Neoliberalism and the contract state: exploring innovation and resistance among New Zealand Health Promoters. *Critical Public Health*, 24(3):308–20.

Lupton, D. (2012) M-health and health promotion: the digital cyborg and surveillance society. *Social Theory and Health*, 10(3):229–44.

Lupton, D. (2013a) *Digitized Health Promotion: Personal Responsibility for Health in the Web 2.0 Era*. Sydney Health & Society Group Working Paper No. 5.

Lupton, D. (2013b) Quantifying the body: monitoring and measuring health in the age of mHealth technologies. *Critical Public Health*, 23:393–403.

Lupton, D. (2014a) The commodification of patient opinion: the digital patient experience economy in the age of big data. *Sociology of Health and Illness*, 36(6):856–69.

Lupton, D. (2014b) How do you measure up? Assumptions about 'obesity' and health-related behaviours and beliefs in two Australian 'obesity' prevention campaigns. *Fat Studies*, 3:32–44.

Lupton, D. (2015a) *Digital Sociology*. London: Routledge.

Lupton, D. (2015b) Quantified sex: a critical analysis of sexual and reproductive self-tracking using apps. *Culture, Health and Sexuality*, 17(4):440–53.

Lupton, D. (2015c) Health promotion in the digital era: a critical commentary. *Health Promotion International*, 30(1):174–83.

MacFadyen, L., Stead, M. and Hastings, G. (1999) *A Synopsis of Social Marketing*. Stirling: Institute for Social Marketing.

Mackenzie, M., Hastings, A., Babbel, B., Simpson, S. and Watt, G. (2017) Tackling and mitigating health inequalities – policymakers and practitioners 'Talk and Draw' their theories. *Social Policy and Administration*, 51(1):151–70.

Mackert, M., Mabry-Flynn, A., Champlin, S., Donovan, E. E. and Pounders, K. (2016) Health literacy and health information technology adoption: the potential for a new digital divide. *Journal of Medical Internet Research*, 18(10):e264.

Magnan, S. (2017) Social determinants of health 101 for health care: five plus five. *NAM Perspectives.* Discussion Paper, National Academy of Medicine, Washington, DC.

Maher, C., Ryan, J., Ambrosi, C. and Edney, S. (2017) Users' experiences of wearable activity trackers: a cross-sectional study. *BMC Public Health*, 17:880.

Mann, H. H. (2006) Empowerment in terms of theoretical perspectives: exploring a typology of the process and components across disciplines. *Journal of Community Psychology*, 34(5):523–40.

Mann, S. and Bailey, J. V. (2016) *Implementation of digital interventions for sexual health for young people.* Frontiers Public Health. Conference Abstract: 2nd Behaviour Change Conference: Digital Health and Wellbeing, London.

Marmot, M. (2010) *Fair Society, Healthy Lives: Strategic Review of Health Inequalities in England Post 2010.* London: Department of Health.

Marschang, S. (2014) *Health Inequalities and eHealth: Report of the eHealth Stakeholders Group.* Brussels: European Public Health Alliance (EPHA).

Martin, S., Sutcliffe, P. Griffiths, F., et al. (2011) Effectiveness and impact of networked communication interventions in young people with mental health conditions: a systematic review. *Patient Education and Counselling*, 85:e108–e119.

Martínez-Pérez, B., Torre-Díez, I. and López-Coronado, M. (2014) Privacy and security in mobile health apps: a review and recommendations. *Journal of Medical System*, 39:181.

Masse, R. and Williams-Jones, B. (2012) Ethical dilemmas in health promotion practice. In I. Rootman, S. Dupere, A. Pederson and M. O'Neill (eds.) *Health Promotion in Canada* (3rd edn.). Toronto: Canadian Scholars.

McElhinney, E., Kidd, L. and Cheater, F. M. (2018) Health literacy practices in social virtual worlds and the influence on health behaviour. *Global Health Promotion*, 25(4): 34–47.

McPhail-Bell, K., Bond, C., Brough, M. and Fredericks, B. (2015) 'We don't tell people what to do': ethical practice and Indigenous health promotion. *Health Promotion Journal of Australia*, 26:195–9.

McQuail, D. (2010) *McQuail's Mass Communication Theory* (6th edn). London: Sage Publications.

McQuail, D. and Windahl, S. (1993) *Communication Models for the Study of Mass Communication* (2nd edn). London: Longman.

Melton, B. F., Bigham, L. E., Bland, H. W., Bird, M. and Fairman, C. (2014) Health-related behaviours and technology usage among college students. *American Journal of Health Behaviour*, 38(4):510–18.

Meyer, B., Bierbrodt, J., Schröder, J., Berger, T., Beeverse, C. G., Weissa, M., et al. (2015) Effects of an Internet intervention (Deprexis) on severe depression symptoms: randomized controlled trial. *Internet Interventions*, 2:48–59.

Meyer, J. H. F., Land, R. and Baillie, C. (2010) *Threshold Concepts and Transformational Learning*. Rotterdam, Boston, Taipei: Sense Publishers.

Mezirow, J. (1997) *Transformative Learning: Theory to Practice*. New Directions for Adult and Continuing Education, no. 74. San Francisco: Jossey-Bass Publications.

Mezirow, J. (2003) Transformative Learning as discourse. *Journal of Transformative Education*, 1:58–63.

Michie, S., Brown, J. Geraghty, A. W. A., Miller, S., Yardley, L., Gardner, B., et al. (2012) Development of StopAdvisor: a theory-based interactive internet-based smoking cessation intervention. *Translational Behavioral Medicine*, 2:263–75.

Mielewczyk, F. and Willig, C. (2007) Old clothes and an older look – the case for a radical makeover in health behaviour research. *Theory and Psychology*, 17(6):811–37.

Miller, T., Chandler, L. and Mouttapa, M. (2015) A needs assessment, development, and formative evaluation of a health promotion smartphone application for college students. *American Journal of Health Education*, 46:207–15.

Miller, P. and Rose, N. (1993) Governing economic life. In M. Gane, and T. Johnson (eds.) *Foucault's New Domains*. London: Routledge.

Milligan, C., Roberts, C. and Mort, M. (2011) Telecare and older people: who cares where? *Social Science and Medicine*, 72: 347–54.

Milne, R.A., Puts, M. T. E., Papadakos, J., Le, L. W., Milne, V.

C., Hope, A. J., et al. (2014) Predictors of high eHealth literacy in primary lung cancer survivors. *Journal of Cancer Education*, 30:685–92.

Miorandi, D., Sicari, S., De Pellegrini, F. and Chlamtac, I. (2012) Internet of things: vision, applications and research challenges. *Ad Hoc Networks*, 10:1497–1516.

Mittelmark, M. B. (2007) Setting an ethical agenda for health promotion. *Health Promotion International*, 23(1):78–85.

Mittelstadt, B. D. and Floridi, L. (2016) The ethics of Big Data: current and foreseeable issues in biomedical contexts. *Science and Engineering Ethics*, 22:303–41.

Mohr, D. C., Duffecy, J., Ho, J., et al. (2013) A randomized controlled trial evaluating a manualized teleCoaching protocol for improving adherence to a Web-based intervention for the treatment of depression. *PLOS ONE*, 8(8):e70086.

Moore, G. E. (1965) Cramming more components onto integrated circuits. *Electronics*, 38(8):114–17.

Moorhead, S. A., Hazlett, D. E., Harrison, L., Carroll, J. K., Irwin, A. and Hoving, C. (2013) A new dimension of health care: systematic review of the uses, benefits, and limitations of social media for health communication. *Journal of Medical Internet Research*, 15(4):e85.

Morin, C. M., Belanger, L. and LeBlanc, M. (2009) The natural history of insomnia: a population-based 3–year longitudinal study. *Archives of Internal Medicine*, 169:447–53.

Morrison, L., Moss-Morris, R., Michie, S. and Yardley, L. (2014) Optimizing engagement with Internet-based health behaviour change interventions: comparison of self-assessment with and without tailored feedback using a mixed methods approach. *British Journal of Health Psychology*, 19:839–55.

Mpongwana, M. (2018, unpublished) The use of electronic systems in dispensing medication for patients with chronic illness in South Africa. Stellenbosch: Stellenbosch University.

Mudge, S., Kayes, N. and McPherson, K. (2015) Who is in control? Clinicians' view on their role in self-management approaches: a qualitative metasynthesis. *BMJ Open*, 5:e007413.

Mwinyuri, V. (2014, unpublished) An evaluation of communication strategies for malaria control in the upper-west region of Ghana during years 2012–2014. Accra: Ghana Health Service.

Naidoo, N. and Wills, J. (2009) *Health Promotion: Foundations for Practice* (3rd edn). London: Baillière Tindall.

Naslund, J. A., Aschbrenner, K. A., Araya, R., et al. (2017) Digital technology for treating and preventing mental disorders in low-income and middle-income countries: a narrative review of the literature. *Lancet Psychiatry*, 4:486–500.

National Audit Office (2013). *Review of the Final Benefits Statement for Programmes Previously Managed under the National Programme for IT in the NHS*. London: National Audit Office.

National Health Service (NHS) (2014) *NHS Five Year Forward View Followed in England*. London: HMSO.

National Health Service (NHS) (2017) *Next Steps on the NHS Five Year Forward View in England*. London: HMSO.

National Health Service (NHS) Choices (2015) *NHS Choices Service Performance*. NHS Choices website.

National Information Board (2014) *Personalised Health and Care: A Framework for Action 2020*. London: HMSO.

National Social Marketing Centre (n.d.) Social Marketing benchmark criteria [online]. Available at www.thensmc.com/resource/social-marketing-benchmark-criteria.

`Neuhauser, L., Kreps, G. L., Morrison, K., Athanasoulis, M., Kirienko, N. and Van Brunt, D. (2013) Using design science and artificial intelligence to improve health communication: ChronologyMD case example. *Patient Education and Counselling*, 92:211–17.

Newman, L., Baum, F., Javanparast, S., O'Rourke, K. and Carlon, L. (2015) Addressing social determinants of health inequities through settings: a rapid review. *Health Promotion International*, 30(S2):ii126–ii143.

NHS Management Executive (1992). *An Information Management and Technology Strategy for England*. London: NHS Management Executive.

Norman, C. (2012) Social media and health promotion. *Global Health Promotion*, 19(4):3–6.

Norman, C. and Skinner, H. (2006) eHealth literacy: essential skills for consumer health in a networked world. *Journal of Medical Internet Research*, 8(2): e9.

Nuffield Council on Bioethics (2007) *Public Health Ethical Issues*. London: Nuffield Council on Bioethics.

Nutbeam, D. (2000) Health literacy as a public health goal: a challenge for contemporary health education and communication strategies into the 21st century. *Health Promotion International*, 15(3):259–67.

Nutbeam, D. (2008) The evolving concept of health literacy. *Social Science and Medicine*, 67(12):2072–8.

Nys, T. R. V. and Engelen, B. (2017) Judge nudging: answering the manipulation objection. *Political Studies*, 65(1):199–214.

O'Dowd, A. (2017) Spending on junk food advertising is nearly 30 times what government spends on promoting healthy eating. *BMJ Open*, 359:j4677.

Ofcom (2014) *Adults' Media Use and Attitudes Report*. London: Ofcom.

Ofcom (2015) *The Communications Market Report*. London: Ofcom.

Office for National Statistics (2014) *Internet Access – Households and Individuals: 2014*. London: Office for National Statistics.

O'Hara, L. and Taylor, J. (2018) What's wrong with the 'war on obesity'? A narrative review of the weight-centered health paradigm and development of the 3C Framework to build critical competency for a paradigm shift. *Sage Open*, 2018:1–28.

O'Hara, L., Taylor, J. and Barnes, M. (2015) The extent to which the public health 'war on obesity' reflects the ethical values and principles of critical health promotion: a multimedia critical discourse analysis. *Health Promotion Journal of Australia*, 26:246–54.

Oliver, A. (2013) From nudging to budging: using behavioural economics to inform public sector policy. *Journal of Social Policy*, 42(4):685–700.

O'Mara, B. (2012) Social media, digital video and health promotion in a culturally and linguistically diverse Australia. *Health Promotion International*, 28(3):466–76.

O'Neil, I. (2008) Public health policy. In J. Mitcheson (ed.) *Public Health Approaches to Practice*. Cheltenham: Nelson Thornes.

Orlowski, S. K., Lawn, S., Venning, A., et al. (2015) Participatory research as one piece of the puzzle: a systematic review of consumer involvement in design of technology-based youth mental health and well-being interventions. *Journal of Medical Internet Research, Human Factors*, 2(2):e12.

Pagoto, S., Schneider, K. L., Evans, M., et al. (2014) Tweeting it off: characteristics of adults who tweet about a weight loss attempt. *Journal of the American Medical Informatics Association*, 21:1032–7.

Paige, S. R., Krieger, J. L., Stellefson, M. and Alber, J. M. (2017) eHealth literacy in chronic disease patients: an item response theory analysis of the eHealth literacy scale (eHEALS). *Patient Education and Counselling*, 100:320–6.

Patel, V., Araya, R., Chatterjee, S., et al. (2007) Treatment and prevention of mental disorders in low-income and middle-income countries. *Lancet*, 370:991–1005.

Patel, V., Maj, M., Flisher, A. J., et al. (2010) Reducing the treatment gap for mental disorders: a WPA survey. *World Psychiatry*, 9:169–76.

Pause, C. (2017) Borderline: the ethics of fat stigma in public health. *Journal of Law, Medicine and Ethics*, 45:510–17.

Petersen, I., Evans-Lacko, S., Semrau, M., et al. (2016) Promotion, prevention and protection: interventions at the population- and community-levels for mental, neurological and substance use disorders in low- and middle-income countries. *International Journal of Mental Health Systems*, 10:30.

Petty, R. and Cacioppo, J. (1986) The elaboration likelihood model of persuasion. *Advanced Experimental Social Psychology*, 19:123–205.

PEW (2016) *Report on Internet Use in 2016*. Washington, DC: PEW Research Centre.

PHPSU (Public Health Policy Strategy Unit) (2015) *Local Authority Public Health Allocations 2015/16: In-year Savings – A consultation*. London, Public Health Policy and Strategy Unit, Department of Health.

Piette, J. D., Lun, K. C., Moura, L. A., et al. (2012) Impacts of e-health on the outcomes of care in low- and middle-income countries: where do we go from here? *Bulletin of the World Health Organization*, 90:332–40.

Pillai, V., Anderson, J. R., Cheng, P., et al. (2015) The anxiolytic effects of cognitive behavior therapy for insomnia: preliminary results from a Web-delivered protocol. *Journal of Sleep Medicine and Disorders*, 2(2):1017.

Piwek, L., Ellis, D. A., Andrews, S. and Joinson, A. (2016) The rise of consumer health wearables: promises and barriers. *PLOS Medicine*, 13(2):1001953.

Pleasant, A., McKinney, J. and Rikard, R. V. (2011) Health literacy measurement: a proposed research agenda. *Journal of Health Communication*, 16:11–21.

Popay, J., Whitehead, M. and Hunter, D. J. (2010) Injustice is killing people on a large scale – but what is to be done about it? *Journal of Public Health*, 32(2):148–9.

Prier, K. W., Smith, M. S., Giraud-Carrier, C. and Hanson, C. L. (2011) Identifying health-related topics on Twitter. In J. Salerno, S. J. Yang, D. Nau and S. K. Chai (eds.) *Social Computing, Behavioural-Cultural Modelling and Prediction*. Lecture Notes in Computer Science. Berlin, Heidelberg: Springer.

Primack, B. A., Carroll, M. V., McNamara, M., et al. (2012) Role of video games in improving health-related outcomes: a systematic review. *American Journal of Preventive Medicine*, 42(6):630–8.

Prochaska, J. O. and DiClemente, C. C. (1984) *The Transtheoretical Approach: Towards a Systematic Eclectic Framework*. Homeward, IL: Dow Jones Irwin.

Public Health England (PHE) (2015) *Sugar Reduction: The Evidence for Action*. London: Public Health England.

Public Health England (PHE) (2016a) *Sexually Transmitted Infections (STIs): Annual Data Tables. 2016*. London: Public Health England.

Public Health England (PHE) (2016b) *Public Health Skills and Knowledge Framework*. London: Public Health England.

Rajatonirina, S., Heraud, J., Randrianasolo, L., et al. (2012) Short message service sentinel surveillance of influenza in Madagascar, 2008–2012. *Bulletin of the World Health Organization*, 90:385–9.

Ramanadhan, S., Mendez, S. R., Rao, M. and Viswanath, K. (2013) Social media use by community-based organizations conducting health promotion: a content analysis. *BMC Public Health*, 13:1129.

Ranard, B. L., Ha, Y. P., Meisel, Z. F. et al. (2013) Crowdsourcing – harnessing the masses to advance health and medicine, a systematic review. *Society of General Internal Medicine*, 29(1):187–203.

Ratzan, S. C. (2011) Our new 'social' communication age in health. *Journal of Health Communication: International Perspectives*, 16(8):803–4.

Raven, B. H. and Litman-Adizes, T. (1986) Interpersonal influence and social power in health promotion. In W. B. Ward (ed.), *Advances in Health Education and Promotion*. London: Elsevier Science Ltd.

Raynor, D. K. (2012) Health literacy. *British Medical Journal online*, 344:e2188.

Ren, W., Huang, C., Liu, Y. and Ren, J. (2017) The application of digital technology in community health education. *Digital Medicine*, 1(1):3–6.

Ricciardi, F. and De Paolis, L.T. (2014) A comprehensive review of serious games in health professions. *International Journal of Computer Games Technology*, Volume 2014, Article ID 787968.

Rice, E., Haynes, E., Royce, P. and Thompson, S. C. (2016) Social media and digital technology use among Indigenous young people in Australia: a literature review. *International Journal for Equity in Health*, 15:81.

Richtering, S. S., Morris, R., Soh, S. E., et al. (2017) Examination of an eHealth literacy scale and a health literacy scale in a population with moderate to high cardiovascular risk. *PLOS ONE*, 12(4):e0175372.

Ritzer, G., Dean, P. and Jurgenson, N. (2012) The coming of age of the prosumer. *American Behavioural Scientist*, 56:379–98.

Roberts, N., Axas, N., Nesdole, R. and Repetti, L. (2016) Pediatric emergency department visits for mental health crisis: prevalence of cyber bullying in suicidal youth. *Child Adolescent Social Work Journal*, 33:469–72.

Rogers, R. W. (1975) A protection motivation theory of fear appeals and attitude change. *Journal of Psychology*, 91:93–114.

Ronit, K. and Jensen, J. D. (2014) Obesity and industry self-regulation of food and beverage marketing: a literature review. *European Journal of Clinical Nutrition*, 68:758.

Rowland, J. L., Malone, L. A., Fidopiastis, C. M., Padalabalanarayanan, S., Thirumalai, M. and Rimmer, J. H. (2016) Perspectives on active video gaming as a new frontier in accessible physical activity for youth with physical disabilities. *Physical Therapy*, 96(4):521–32.

Royal College of Paediatrics and Child Health (RCPCH) (2018) RCPCH responds to Lancet findings on recreational screen time. *Royal College of Paediatrics and Child Health* [online]. Available at www.rcpch.ac.uk/news-events/news/rcpch-responds-lancet-findings-recreational-screen-time.

Rutter, M. (1980). *Changing Youth in a Changing Society. Patterns of Adolescent Development and Disorder.* London: Harvard University Press.

Saberi, P., Siedle-Khan, R., Sheon, N. and Lightfoot, M. (2016) The use of mobile health applications among youth and young adults living with HIV: Focus Group findings. *AIDs Patient Care and STDs*, 30(6):254-2-60.

Salas, X. R. (2015) The ineffectiveness and unintended consequences of the public health war on obesity. *Canadian Public Health*, 106(2):e79–e81.

Sanders, C., Rogers, A., Bowen, R., et al. (2012) 'Exploring barriers to participation and adoption of telehealth and telecare within the Whole System Demonstrator trial: a qualitative study', *BMC Health Services Research*, 12:220.

Santos, A., Macedo, J., Costa, A. and Nicolau, M. J. (2014) Internet of Things and smart objects for m-Health monitoring and control. *Procedia Technology*, 16:1351–60.

Saraceno, B., Van Ommeren, M., Batniji, R., et al. (2007) Barriers to improvement of mental health services in low-income and middle-income countries. *Lancet*, 370:1164–74.

Sarkar, U., Karter, A. J. and Liu, J. Y. (2011) Social disparities in Internet patient portal use in diabetes: evidence that the digital divide extends beyond access. *Journal of American Medical Informatics Association*, 18(3):318–21.

Sawesi S., Rashrash, M., Phalakornkule, K., Carpenter, J. S. and Jones, J. F. (2016) The impact of information technology on patient engagement and health behaviour change: a systematic review of the literature. *Journal of Medical Internet Research*, 4(1):e1.

Scanfeld, D., Scanfeld, V. and Larson, E. L. (2010) Dissemination of health information through social networks: Twitter and anti-biotics. *American Journal of Infection Control*, 38(3):182–8.

Schramm, W. (1954) How communication works. In D. McQuail and S. Windahl (ed.) (1993) *Communication Models for the Study of Mass Communications* (2nd edn). London: Longman.

Schwind, J. S., Norman, S. A., Karmacharya, D., et al. (2017) Online surveillance of media health event reporting in Nepal:

digital disease detection from a One Health perspective. *BMC International Health and Human Rights*, 17:26.

Scott-Samuel, A. and Smith, K. E. (2015) Fantasy paradigms of health inequalities: Utopian thinking? *Social Theory and Health*, 13(3–4):418–36.

Scottish Government (2013) *Digital Scotland 2020: Achieving World-Class Digital Infrastructure: A Final Report to The Scottish Government*. Edinburgh: The Scottish Government.

Seedhouse, D. (2001) *The Foundations for Achievement* (2nd edn). Chichester: John Wiley and Sons.

Seidenberg, P., Nicholson, S., Schaefer, M., et al. (2012) Early infant diagnosis of HIV infection in Zambia through mobile phone texting of blood test results. *Bulletin of the World Health Organization*, 90:348–56.

Semkovska, M. and Ahern, E. (2017) Online neurocognitive remediation therapy to improve cognition in community-living individuals with a history of depression: a pilot study. *Internet Interventions*, 9:7–14.

Shah, S. G. S., Fitton, R., Hannan, A., Fisher, B., Young, T. and Barnett, J. (2015) Accessing personal medical records online: a means to what ends? *International Journal of Medical Informatics*, 84:111–18.

Shannon, C. and Weaver, W. (1949) The mathematical theory of communication. In D. McQuail and S. Windahl (eds.) (1993) *Communication Models for the Study of Mass Communication* (2nd edn). London: Longman.

Shet, A., Arumugam, K., Rodrigues, R., Rajagopalan, N., Shubha, K., Raj, T., et al. (2010) Designing a mobile phone-based intervention to promote adherence to Antiretroviral therapy in South India. *AIDS Behaviour*, 14:716–20.

Silva, S., Badasyan, N. and Busby, M. (2018) Diversity and digital divide: using the National Broadband Map to identify the non-adopters of broadband. *Telecommunications Policy*, 42:361–73.

Simons, M., Chinapaw, M. J., van de Bovenkamp, M., et al. (2014) Active video games as a tool to prevent excessive weight gain in adolescents: rationale, design and methods of a randomized controlled trial. *BMC Public Health*, 14:275.

Sindall, C. (2002) Does health promotion need a code of ethics? *Health Promotion International*, 17(3):201–3.

Skinner, H. A., Maley, O. and Norman, C. D. (2006) Developing Internet-based eHealth promotion programs: the Spiral Technology Action Research (STAR) model. *Health Promotion Practice*, 7(4):406–17.

Sleep Council (2011) *Toxic Sleep: The Silent Epidemic*. Skipton: Sleep Council.

Sorensen, K., Karuranga, S., Denysiuk, E. and McLernon, L. (2018) Health literacy and social change: exploring networks and interest groups shaping the rising global health literacy movement. *Global Health Promotion*, 25(4):89–92.

Sorensen, K., van den Broucke, S., Fulham, J., et al. (2012) Health literacy and public health: a systematic review and integration of definitions and models. *BMC Public Health*, 12:80.

Staples, L. H. (1990). Powerful ideas about empowerment. *Administration in Social Work*, 14(2):29–42.

Stellefson, M., Paige, S. R., Tennant, B., et al. (2017) Reliability and validity of the Telephone-Based eHealth Literacy Scale among older adults: cross-sectional survey. *Journal of Medical Internet Research*, 19(10):e362.

Stephenson, A., McDonough, S., Murphy, M. H., Nugent, C. D. and Mair, J. L. (2017) Using computer, mobile and wearable technology enhanced interventions to reduce sedentary behaviour: a systematic review and meta-analysis. *International Journal of Behavioural Nutrition and Physical Activity*, 14:105.

Stevenson, F.A., Kerr, C., Murray, E., and Nazareth, I. (2007) Information from the Internet and the doctor–patient relationship: the patient perspective – a qualitative study. *BMC Family Practice*, 8.

Steventon, A., Tunkel, S., Blunt, I. and Bardsley, M. (2013) Effect of telephone health coaching (Birmingham OwnHealth) on hospital use and associated costs: cohort study with matched controls. *British Medical Journal* 347, f4585.

Sugden, R. (2009) On Nudge: a review of Nudge: Improving Decisions about Health, Wealth and Happiness by Richard H. Thaler and Cass R. Sunstein. *International Journal of the Economics of Business*, 16(3):365–73.

Swan, M. (2012) Crowdsourced health research studies: an important emerging complement to clinical trials in the public health research ecosystem. *Journal of Medical Internet Research*, 14(2):e46.

Sweeney, G. M., Donovan, C. L., March, S. and Forbes, Y. (2019) Logging into therapy: adolescent perceptions of online therapies for mental health problems. *Internet Interventions*, 15:93–9.

Sykes, S. and Wills, J. (2018) Challenges and opportunities in building critical health literacy. *Global Health Promotion*, 25(4):48–56.

Tarouco, L. M. R., Bertholdo, L. M., Granville, L. Z., et al. (2012) *Internet of Things in Healthcare: Interoperability and Security Issues. IEEE International Conference on Communications.* Ottawa: IEEE.

Techcrunch (2017) Report by Constine J. on monthly users on internet sites. Available at: https://techcrunch.com/2017/06/27/facebook-2-billion-users.

Telford, L. (1998) Ethical dilemmas in health promotion. *Ontario Health Promotion E-Bulletin*, 79.

Thackeray, R., Neiger, B. L., Hanson, C. and McKenzie, J. F. (2008) Enhancing promotional strategies within social marketing programs: use of Web 2.0 social media. *Health Promotion Practice*, 9:338.

Thackeray, R., Neiger, B. L. and Keller, H. (2012) Integrating social media and social marketing: a four-step process. *Health Promotion Practice*, 13(2):165—8.

Thaler, C. R. and Sunstein, R. H. (2008) *Nudge: Improving Decisions about Health, Wealth and Happiness.* New Haven: Yale University Press.

Thirumurthy, H. and Lester, R. (2012) M-health for health behaviour change in resource-limited settings: applications to HIV care and beyond. *Bulletin of the World Health Organization*, 90:390–2.

Thompson, L. and Kumar, A. (2011) Responses to health promotion campaigns: resistance, denial and othering. *Critical Public Health*, 21:105–17.

Topooco, N., Riper, H., Araya, R., et al. (2017) Attitudes towards digital treatment for depression: a European stakeholder survey. *International Interventions*, 8:1–9.

Tozun, M. and Babaoglu, A. B. (2017) Cyber bullying and its effects on the adolescent and youth health: a huge problem behind tiny keys. *Journal of Clinical and Analytical Medicine*, 9(2):177–82.

Trezona, A., Dodson, S., Mech, P. and Osborne, R. H. (2018)

Development and testing of a framework for analysing health literacy in public health documents. *Global Health Promotion*, 25(4):24–33.

United Nations (2011) *Prevention and Control of Non-communicable Diseases: Report of the Secretary General.* New York: United Nations General Assembly.

United Nations (2015) *The Sustainable Development Goals 2015–2030.* NewYork: United Nations.

US Congressional Committee (1996) Health Insurance Portability and Accountability Act (HIPAA) 1996. Washington, DC: US Government Publishing Office.

US Department of Commerce (2013) *Exploring the Digital Nation.* Washington, DC: US Department of Commerce.

Vallgarda, S. (2012) Nudge – a new and better way to improve health? *Health Policy*, 104:200–3.

Van De Belt, T. H., Engelen, L. J. L. P. G., Berben, S. A. A. and Schoonhoven, L. (2010) Definition of Health 2.0 and Medicine 2.0: a systematic review. *Journal of Medical Internet Research*, 12(2):e18.

Van den Broucke, S. (2014) Health literacy: a critical concept for public health. *Archives of Public Health*, 72:10.

Van Gemert-Pijnen, J., Wynchank, S. and Ossebaard, H. C. (2012) Improving the credibility of electronic health technologies. *Bulletin of the World Health Organization*, 90:323–323A.

Van Heerden, A., Tomlinson, M. and Swartz, L. (2012) Point of care in your pocket: a research agenda for the field of m-health. *Bulletin of the World Health Organization*, 90:393–4.

Veitch, K. (2010) The government of health care and the politics of patient empowerment: New Labour and the NHS reform agenda in England. *Law & Policy*, 32:313–31.

VicHealth (2013) *Fair Foundations: The VicHealth Framework for Health Equity* [online]. Available at www.vichealth.vic.gov.au/media-and-resources/publications/the-vichealth-framework-for-health-equity.

Vos, T., Barber, R. M., Bell, B., Bertozzi-Villa, A., Biryukov, S., Bolliger, I., et al. (2015) Global, regional, and national incidence, prevalence, and years lived with disability for 301 acute and chronic diseases and injuries in 188 countries, 1990–2013: a systematic analysis for the Global Burden of Disease Study 2013. *Lancet*, 386 (9995):743–800.

Wachter, R. M. (2016) *Making IT work: Harnessing the Power of Health Information Technology to Improve Care in England.* London: National Advisory Group on Health Information Technology in England.

Wakefield, M. A., Loken, B. and Hornik R. C. (2010) Use of mass media campaigns to change health behaviour. *Lancet,* 376:1261–71.

Wang, J.-Y., Bennett, K. and Probst, J. (2011) Subdividing the digital divide: differences in internet access and use among rural residents with medical limitations. *Journal of Medical Internet Research*, 13(1):e25.

Waterson, P. (2014) Health information technology and socio-technical systems: a progress report on recent developments within the UK National Health Services. *Applied Ergonomics,* 45:150–61.

Watt, R. G. (2002) Emerging theories into the social determinants of health: implications for oral health promotion. *Community Dentistry and Oral Epidemiology*, 30:241–7.

Webb, T. L. Joseph, J., Yardley, L. and Michie, S. (2010) Using the Internet to promote health behaviour change: a systematic review and meta-analysis of the impact of theoretical basis, use of behaviour change techniques, and mode of delivery on efficacy. *Journal of Medical Internet Research*, 12(1):e4.

Weinreich, N. K. (2006) *What is Social Marketing?* Los Angeles: Weinreich Communications.

Weymann, N., Harter, M. and Dirmaier, J. (2014) Quality of online information on type 2 diabetes: a cross-sectional study. *Health Promotion International*, 30 (4):821–31.

White, D. S. and Le Cornu, A. (2011) Visitors and residents: a new typology for online engagement [online]. *First Monday*, 16(9). Available at: firstmonday.org/article/view/3171/3049.

Whitehead, M. and Popay, J. (2010) Swimming upstream? Taking action on the social determinants of health inequalities. *Sociology of Social Science and Medicine*, 71:1234–6.

Whiting, A. and Williams, D. (2013) Why people use social media: a uses and gratifications approach. *Qualitative Market Research: An International Journal*, 16(4):362–9.

WHO (World Health Organization) (1946) *Constitution of*

the World Health Organization. Copenhagen: World Health Organization.

WHO (World Health Organization) (1978) *Declaration of Alma Ata*. Geneva: World Health Organization.

WHO (World Health Organization) (1981) *Global Strategy for Health for All by the Year 2000*. Geneva: World Health Organization.

WHO (World Health Organization) (1984) *Health Promotion: A Discussion Document on the Concept and Principles: Summary Report of the Working Group on Concept and Principles of Health Promotion*. Copenhagen: World Health Organization.

WHO (World Health Organization) (1986) *Ottawa Charter for Health Promotion*. Copenhagen: World Health Organization.

WHO (World Health Organization) (1988) *The Adelaide Recommendations: Healthy Public Policy*. Geneva: World Health Organization and the Commonwealth of Australia.

WHO (World Health Organization) (1991) *Third International Conference on Health Promotion*. Sundsvall, Sweden and Geneva: World Health Organization.

WHO (World Health Organization) (1997) *Jakarta Declaration on Leading Health Promotion into the 21st Century*. Geneva: World Health Organization.

WHO (World Health Organization) (2000) *Mexico Ministerial Statement for the Promotion of Health: From Ideas to Action. Fifth Global Conference on Health Promotion: Bridging the Equity Gap*. Mexico, Geneva: World Health Organization.

WHO (World Health Organization) (2005a) *eHealth: Resolution and Decisions*. World Health Assembly (WHA) 58.28. Geneva: World Health Organization.

WHO (World Health Organization) (2005b) *The Bangkok Charter for Health Promotion in a Global World*. Geneva: World Health Organization.

WHO (World Health Organization) (2008) *Closing the Gap in a Generation: Health Equity Through Action on the Social Determinants of Health. Final Report of the Commission on Social Determinants of Health*. Geneva: World Health Organization.

WHO (World Health Organization) (2009) *World Health Organization 7th Global Conference in Nairobi*. Geneva: World Health Organization.

WHO (World Health Organization) (2010) *A Conceptual Framework for Action on the Social Determinants of Health*. Discussion Paper Series on Social Determinants of Health, no. 2. Copenhagen: World Health Organization.

WHO (World Health Organization) (2011a) *mHealth: New Horizons for Health through Mobile Technologies*. Global Observatory for eHealth series, no.3. Geneva: World Health Organization.

WHO (World Health Organization) (2011b) *Social Determinants of Health*. Geneva: World Health Organization.

WHO (World Health Organization) (2012) *World Health Day 2012 – Ageing and Health*. Geneva: World Health Organization.

WHO (World Health Organization) (2013) *Health Literacy*. Copenhagen: World Health Organization.

WHO (World Health Organization) (2014) *Protecting Children from the Harmful Effects of Food and Drink Marketing* [online]. World Health Organization. Available at www.who. int/features/2014/uk-food-drink-marketing/en.

WHO (World Health Organization) (2015) *The European Health Report 2015. Targets and Beyond – Reaching New Frontiers in Evidence. Highlights*. Copenhagen: World Health Organization.

WHO (World Health Organization) (2016) *9th Global Conference for Health Promotion: Shanghai Declaration on Promoting Health in the 2030 Agenda for Sustainable Development*. Copenhagen: World Health Organization.

WHO (World Health Organization) (2017a) *Tracking Universal Health Coverage: 2017 Global Monitoring Report*. Copenhagen: World Health Organization.

WHO (World Health Organization) (2017b) *Assessing and Managing Children at Primary Healthcare Facilities to Prevent Overweight and Obesity in the Context of the Double Burden of Malnutrition*. Copenhagen: World Health Organization.

WHO (World Health Organization) (2017c) *Ten Years in Public Health 2007–2017*. Copenhagen: World Health Organization.

Wilkinson, T. M. (2013) Nudging and manipulation. *Political Studies*, 61:341–55.

Williams, R. (1983) Concepts of health: an analysis of lay logic. *Sociology*, 17:185–204.

Williamson, D. L. and Carr, J. (2009) Health as a resource for everyday life: advancing the conceptualization. *Critical Public Health*, 19(1):107–22.

Winter, S. J., Sheats, J. L. and King, A. (2016) The use of behaviour change technologies and theory in technologies for cardiovascular disease prevention and treatment in adults: a comprehensive review. *Progress in Cardiovascular Diseases*, 58:605–12.

Wootton, R., Geissbuhler, A., Jethwani, K., et al. (2012) Long-running telemedicine networks delivering humanitarian services: experience, performance and scientific output. *Bulletin of the World Health Organization*, 90:341–347D.

World Bank (2016) *World Development Report 2016: Digital Dividends*. Washington, DC: World Bank Group.

Yale Rudd Centre (2013) *Measuring Progress in Nutrition and Marketing to Children and Teens*. Hartford, CT: Yale Rudd Centre for Food Policy and Obesity.

Yank, V., Agarwal, S., Loftus, P., Asch, S. and Rehkopf, D. (2017) Crowdsourced health data: comparability to a US national survey, 2013–2015. *American Journal of Public Health*, 107(8):1283–9.

Zach, L., Dalrymple, P. W., Rogers, M. L. and Williver-Farr, H. (2011) Assessing internet access and use in a medically under-served population: implications for providing enhanced health information services. *Health Information and Libraries Journal*, 29:61–71.

Zimmerman, M. A. (2000) Empowerment theory. In J. Rappaport and E. Seidman (eds.) *Handbook of Community Psychology*. Boston, MA, Springer.

Index

Note: page numbers in *italics* denote boxes, figures or tables

Etkin, J. 23
Europe
  data protection 125
  depression treatment 23
  eHealth 140
  gaming 39
  Health 2020 102
  health literacy 143–4
  medical records 109
  social determinants 128
  see also specific countries
European Health 106
European Health Literacy Consortium
  143–4
European Health Report 2015 128
European Union, GDPR 102, 125
Evidence Centre, The 17
evidence-based practice 35, 131,
  157–8, 159, 164, 168
exercise 36, 37
exergames 37, 38
expert patients 153–4
experts – information receivers 47–8
exploitation 70, 153
Exploring the Digital Nation, USA
  139
extrinsic rewards 22

Facebook 3, 14, 25, 29, 101, 115,
  122
Facebook Messenger 115
FaceSpace 30
face-tracking technology 24
Fair Foundations (VicHealth) 63
Fair Society, Healthy Lives (Marmot)
  130
family planning 28, 92
Farnell, G. 23
Federal Trade Commission Act 125
feedback 24, 48, 76, 80–2, 89
Fernández-Aranda, F. 39
fertility management 28
Fishbein, M. 85, 86–7
Fisher, M. 135–6
Fitbits 12, 23, 67
fitness 21, 39, 53, 75–6, 77, 157
Fletcher, S. 31–2

Floridi, L. 123, 124
'Flu Near You' 118
food advertising 79–80, 136–7
Food Foundation, The 136
Foucault, M. 68, 73, 78, 116
Free, C. 18–19
free-market choices 77, 130, 143–4
Freire, P. 32, 51
Frohlich, K. L. 152

gamification 7, 12, 22, 24, 35–40
GDPR (General Data Protection
  Regulation) 125
gender differences
  behaviour approach 95
  cyberbullying 112–13
  Facebook users 115
  fertility management 28
  internet use/access 3, 135
  mobile phone use 150
  SDGs 103
  text messaging 151
  violence against 38, 102
General Data Protection Regulation
  (GDPR) 125
generalized resistance resources
  (GRRs) 152–3
genome sequencing 6
Ghana 16, 35
Gibbons, M. C. 154, 155
Glasheen, K. J. 33
Global Health Promotion 46
Global North/South 14–15, 82–3,
  100–1, 156
globalization
  Big Data 7, 43, 101, 126
  consumerism 14, 43
  mHealth 125
  neoliberalism 14, 43
  public health 101, 103
  social media 112–13
Gold, J. 28, 30, 31
Good Things Foundation 148
Goodwin, T. 41, 134
Google Android 20, 124–5
Google Play 21
Gordon, R. 94–5